Cancer Friendly Cookbook

The Very Best 30 Cancer Friendly Recipes

BY

MOLLY MILLS

Copyright © 2020 by Molly Mills

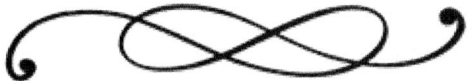

License Notes

No part of this book may be copied, replicated, distributed, sold or shared without the express and written consent of the Author.

The ideas expressed in the book are for entertainment purposes. The Reader assumes all risk when following any guidelines and the Author accepts no responsibility if damages occur due to actions taken by the Reader.

Table of Contents

Introduction 6

Cancer friendly Breakfast ideas 7

    1. Fruity Almond Milk Oatmeal 8

    2. Anti-Inflammation Green Juice 10

    3. Spinach Omelet 12

    4. Vegetable Frittata 14

    5. Flaxseed Orange Muffins 16

    6. Cheesy Avocado Toast 18

    7. Strawberry Buckwheat Porridge 20

    8. Oats Veggie Pancake 22

    9. Spiced Quinoa 24

    10. Scrambled Egg with Broccoli 27

    11. Coconut Carrot Porridge 29

Smoothies 31

    12. Blueberry Orange Smoothie with Muffin 32

    13. Avocado Broccoli Smoothie 34

14. Watermelon Smoothie 36

15. Ginger Carrot Beet Smoothie 38

Soups 40

16. Scallion Asparagus Soup 41

17. Onion Butternut Squash Soup 44

18. Apple Carrot Soup 46

19. Red Lentil Soup 48

20. Pea Vegetable Soup 50

Main course meals 52

21. Cauliflower, Broccoli and Tofu 53

22. Black Beans Vegetable Casserole 55

23. Lamb Cutlets with Mashed Potatoes, Garlic and Peas 58

24. Lentil Dhal with Rice 61

25. Noodles with Ginger and Peanut Sauce 63

26. Salmon with Faro and Caponata 65

27. Chicken with green veggies 68

28. Chicken with Roast Sweet Potatoes 71

29. Chorizo with pea soup 73

30. Stuffed Sweet Potato with Hummus and Beans 75

Conclusion 77

About the Author 78

Don't Miss Out! 79

Introduction

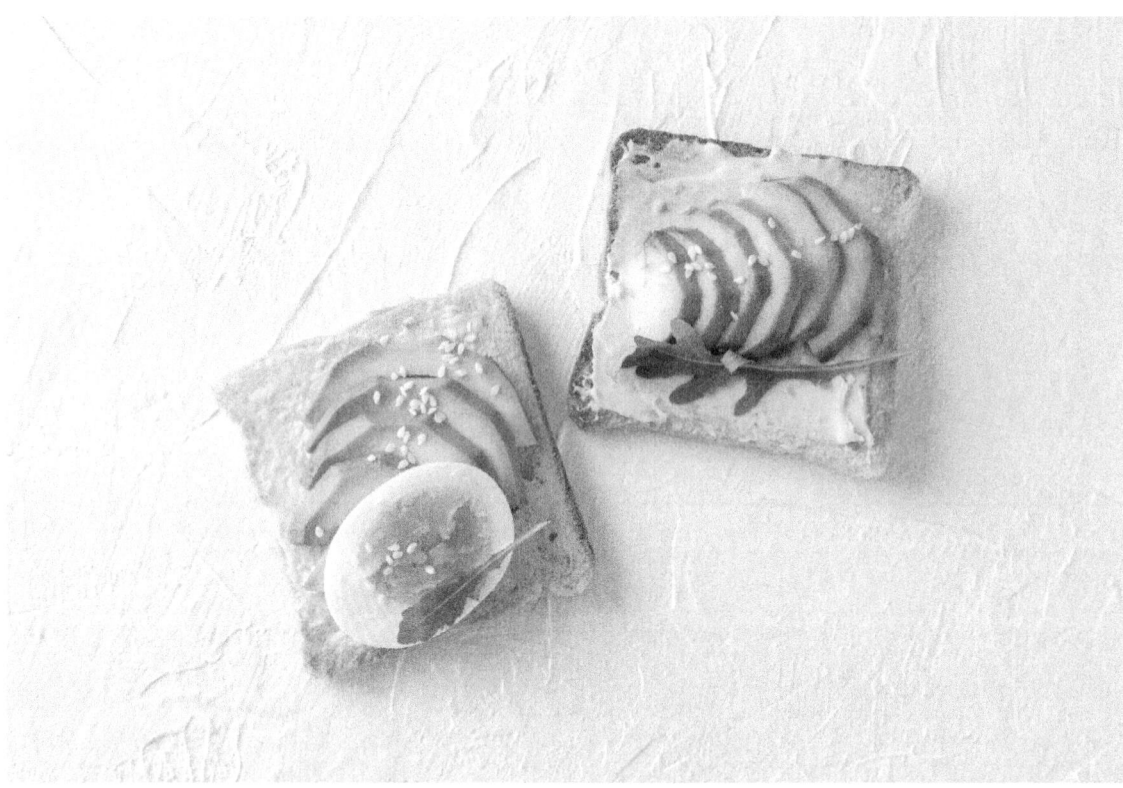

Cancer tends to destroy cells and body tissues, and it is, therefore, necessary to consume enough proteins that help in rejuvenating them. In addition, vegetables and fruits contain fiber and vitamin C, which aid in digestion and boost immunity. Besides, they are packed with antioxidants that help to fight cancer.

To eliminate nausea and loss of appetite, we have incorporated smoothies and juices that are packed with antioxidants, fiber, and curd protein to keep you energized. Try out on our hearty yet easy to prepare recipes, and you will love them.

Enjoy!

Cancer friendly Breakfast ideas

1. Fruity Almond Milk Oatmeal

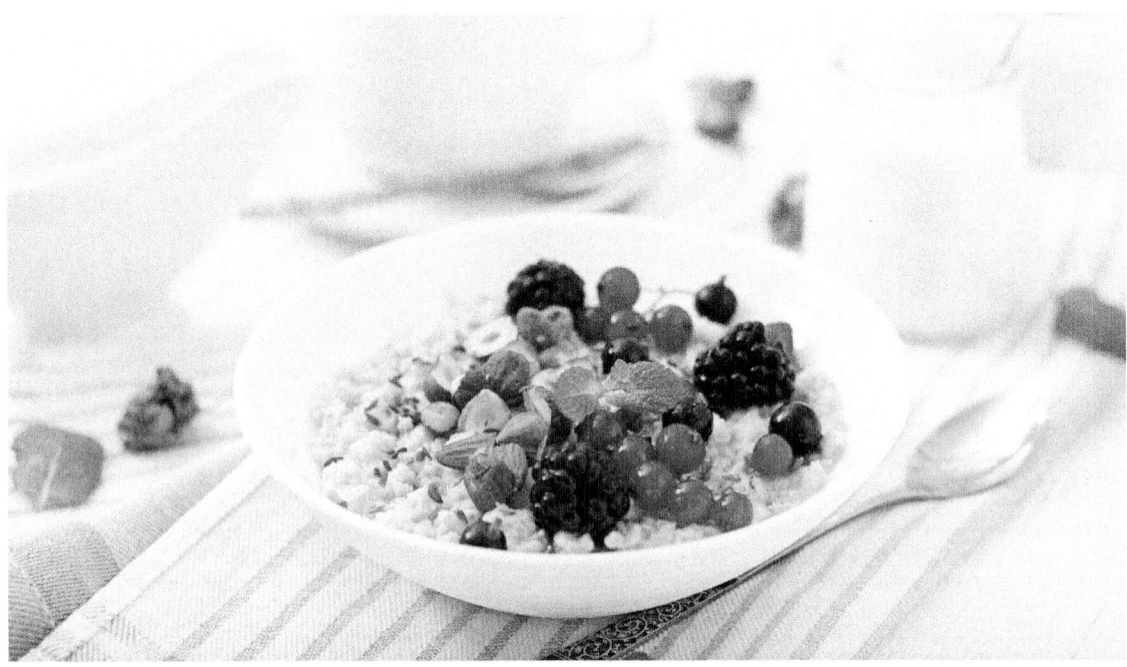

An amazing healthy breakfast that is rich in proteins to help in rejuvenating body cells and decrease the chances of other infections. Besides, the nuts contain omega-3 fatty acids to aid in reducing inflammation and fight the cancer cells. Try out on this easy to make breakfast and benefit from its nutritional value.

Preparation time: 8 minutes **Number of servings:** 1

Ingredients

- 1 teaspoon of chia seeds
- ¼ cup of chopped apple
- 1 tablespoon of finely chopped dates
- ½ cup of rolled oats
- 1 cup of almond milk
- 1 tablespoon of peanut butter
- 1 teaspoon of maple syrup

Preparation method

Add oats, milk, pea butter and maple syrup into a jar and whisk

Stir in the dates and chia seeds

Cork the jar and refrigerate the content for at least 4 hours

Top with apples and serve

2. Anti-Inflammation Green Juice

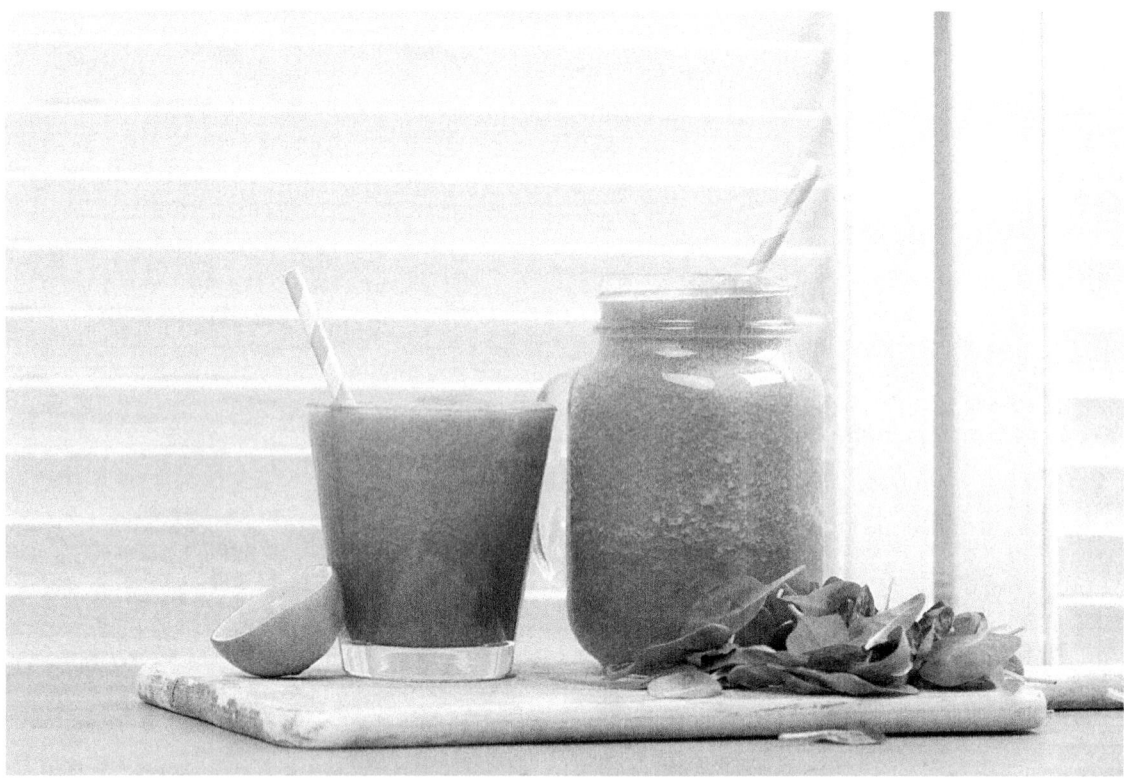

Try out on this green juice full of powerful antioxidants that help fight cancerous cells and suppress the growth of a tumour. Besides, the spinach is rich in minerals and vitamins that will help to boost your immune system. This juice tastes awesome when chilled.

Preparation time: 8 minutes **Number of servings:** 3

Ingredients

- ½ cup of roughly chopped spinach
- ½ teaspoon of apple cider vinegar
- ¾ cup of chopped tomatoes
- 1 ½ cups of chilled water

Preparation method

Into a blender, add the spinach, tomatoes, vinegar, and water

Blend for at least 3 minutes until smooth

Serve the juice into 3 glasses and enjoy

3. Spinach Omelet

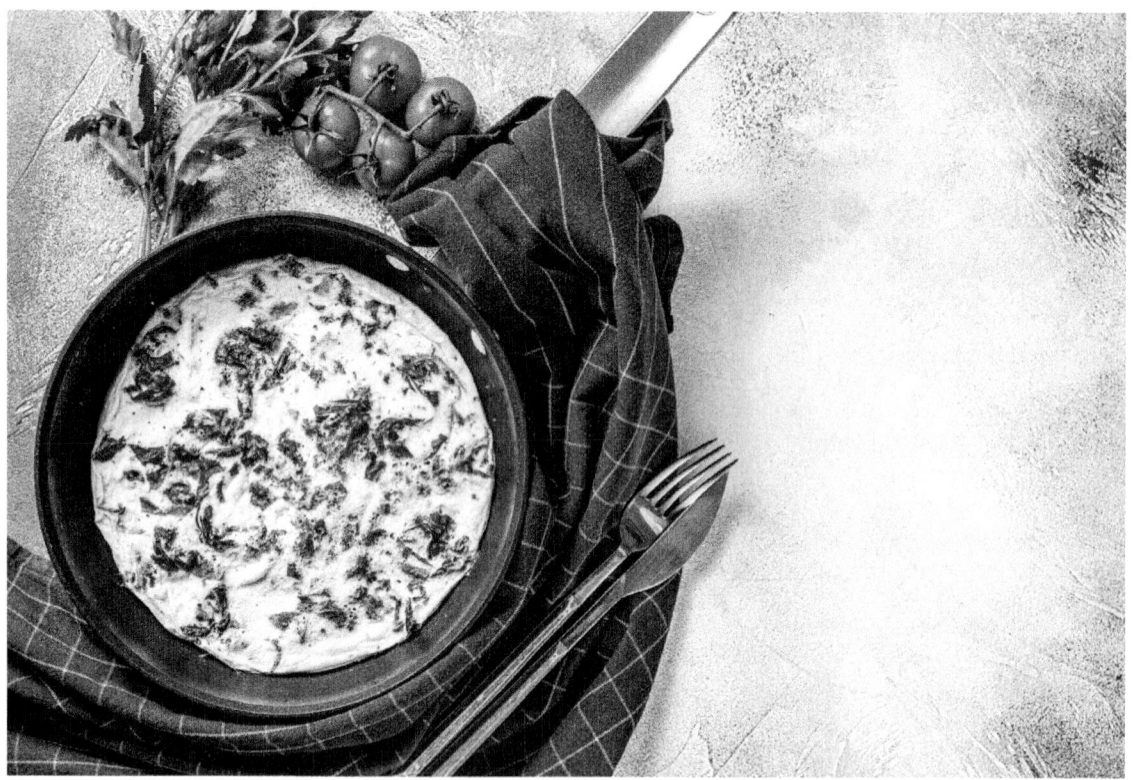

Try out on our spinach omelet recipe that full of antioxidants and an amazing balance of flavours. Besides, it has enough proteins to help in repairing destroyed cells. It is easy to prepare, and you can omit the garlic though it pairs well with spinach. For a dairy-free breakfast, you can replace the milk and cheese with water and grated tofu, respectively.

Preparation time: 15 minutes **Number of servings:** 1

Ingredients

- 2 eggs
- 1 teaspoon of olive oil
- ½ teaspoon of chili flakes (optional)
- 2 minced garlic cloves
- 2 tablespoons of grated parmesan cheese
- 1 tablespoon of skimmed milk
- 1 cup of chopped spinach leaves
- Salt

Preparation method

Into a bowl, crack in the eggs, add the milk, a pinch of salt and whisk well

In a skillet, fry the spinach and garlic until it just wilts and set aside

Into a clean pan, add the oil, pour in the egg mixture, and cook it over medium heat. Once it begins to set, top it up with spinach and sprinkle with grated cheese

Minimize the heat and cook further until the cheese melts

Gently place the omelette on a platter and serve

4. Vegetable Frittata

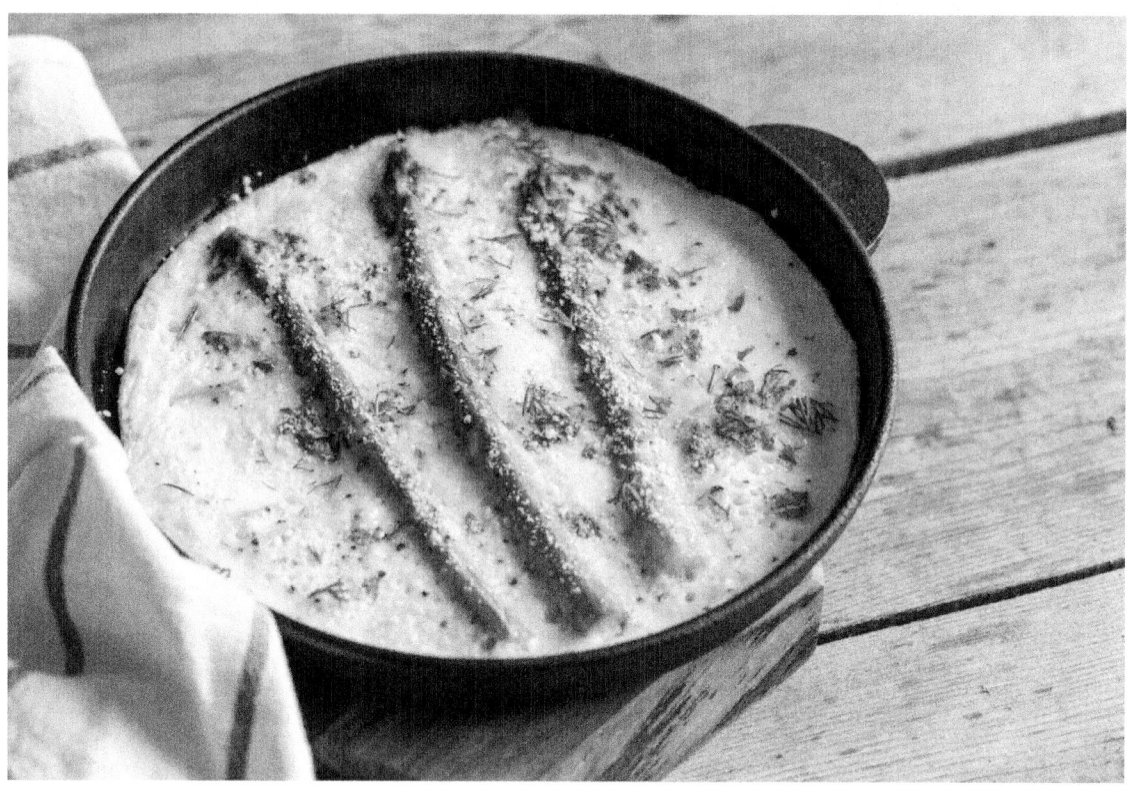

Are you looking for an ideal recipe for patients on a low microbial diet? Try out on our Vegetable frittata recipe that is not only nutritious but also easy to prepare. Besides, it is rich in proteins and vitamins to boost the immune system and energize the body.

Preparation time: 25 minutes **Number of servings:** 6

Ingredients

- ¾ cup of chopped onions
- 5 eggs
- 1 tablespoon of olive oil
- ½ cup of peeled, cooked and diced red potatoes
- 1 tablespoon of chopped parsley
- ½ cup of grated parmesan cheese
- ½ cup of asparagus, diagonally cut into 1- inch pieces
- Salt and ground black pepper

Preparation method

Into a bowl, whisk in the eggs, parsley, cheese, some salt and pepper

Heat the oil over medium heat in a skillet, add the onions, asparagus, and cook-stir them for about 5 minutes until the onions are soft and translucent

Reduce the heat, add in the potatoes and the egg mixture (do not stir)

Cook on low for about 15 minutes until the egg sets

Preheat the broiler and place the skillet under it for about 30 seconds to cook the top of the frittata

Serve and enjoy

5. Flaxseed Orange Muffins

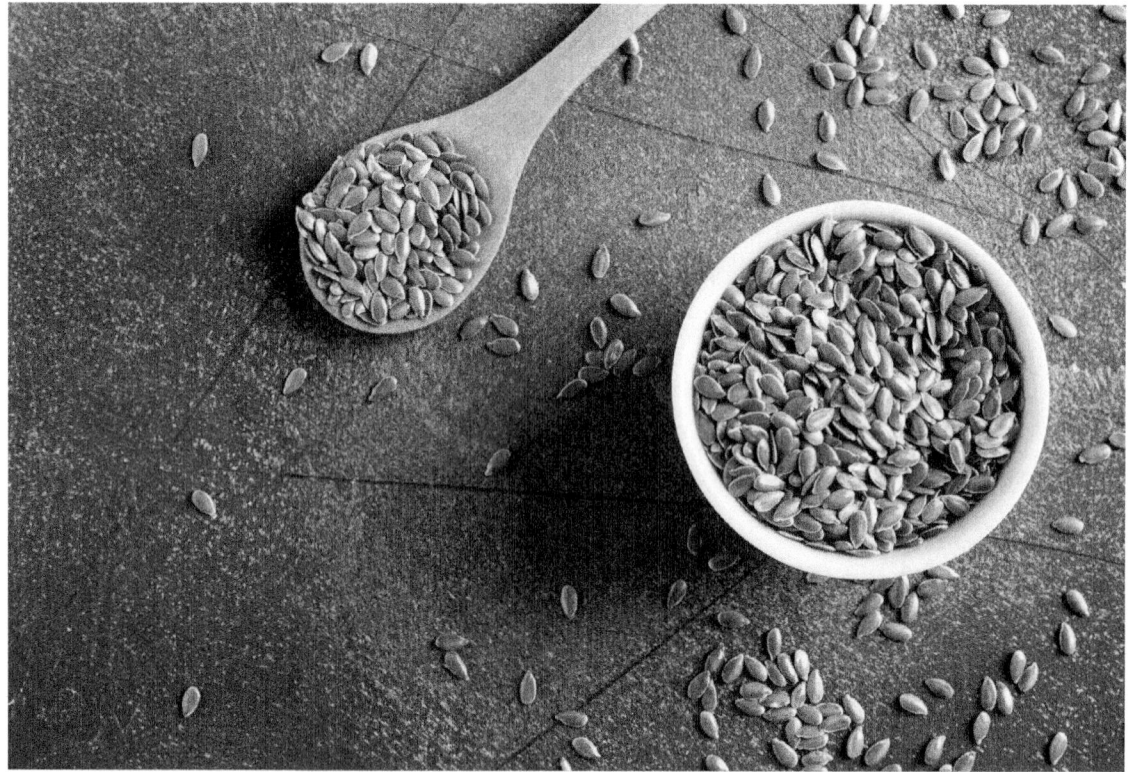

An ideal breakfast for patients on a low microbial diet that you can try on. It is protein-rich, and the flaxseeds contain an omega-3 fatty acid that helps to fight cancer and reduce inflammation. You can substitute the raisins with milk or white chocolate chips, and the taste will be great.

Preparation time: 20 minutes **Number of servings:** 9

Ingredients

- ¾ cup of oat bran
- ½ cup of all-purpose flour
- ½ cup of natural bran
- ½ cup of flaxseed
- ¼ teaspoon of salt
- ½ tablespoon of baking powder
- 2 eggs
- ¾ cup of raisins
- 1 seedless and quartered orange
- ¼ cup of canola oil
- ½ cup of brown sugar
- ½ cup of buttermilk
- ½ teaspoon of baking soda

Preparation method

Into a bowl, combine the oat bran, flaxseeds, flour, baking powder, bran, salt and set the mixture aside

Into a food processor, add the oranges, baking soda sugar, oil, eggs, and pulse until smooth

Pour the orange mixture into the oat bran mixture and combine well

Stir in the raisins and fill the paper-lined muffin tins with the batter

Bat at 3750F for about 20 minutes or until ready

Serve and enjoy

6. Cheesy Avocado Toast

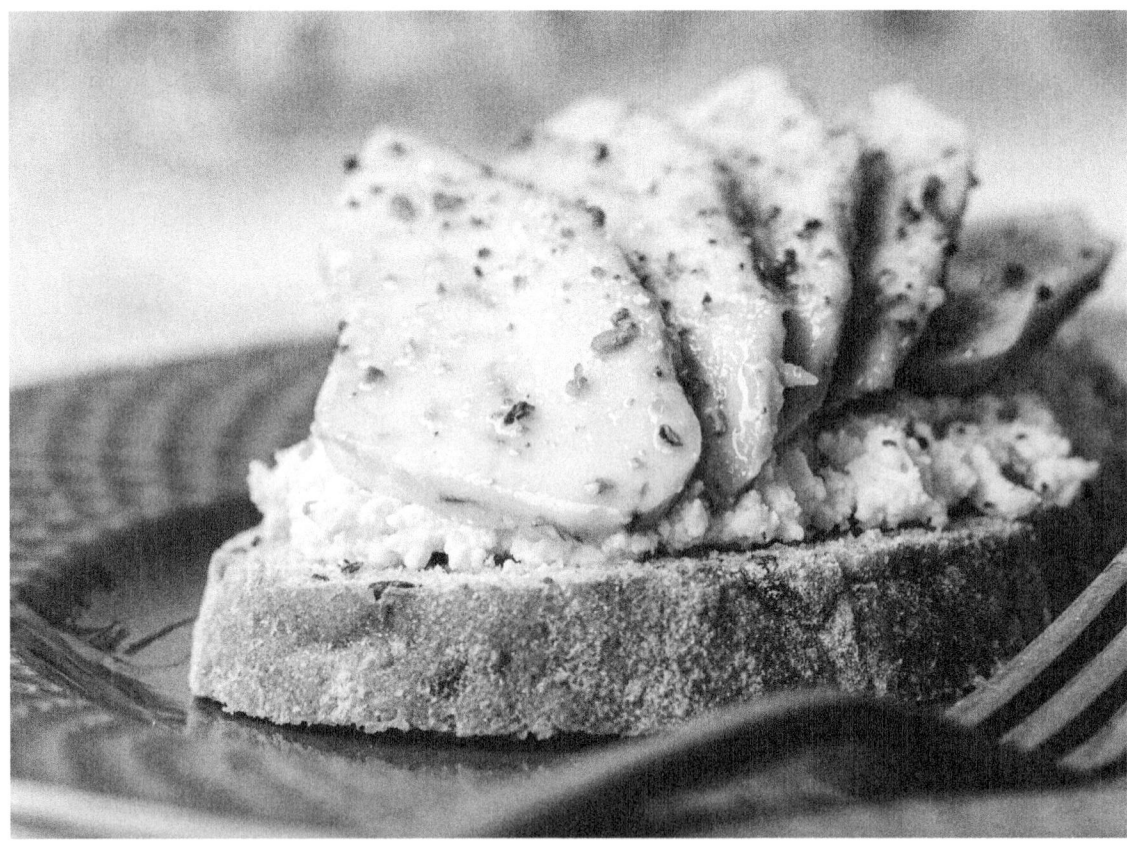

Try out on our flavorful cheesy avocado toast, with loads of healthy **Ingredients** to help fight the cancerous cells. You can serve this toast for breakfast or as a snack for mid-morning. The toast is easy to make, and it will be on your plate within 15 minutes.

Preparation time: 20 minutes **Number of servings:** 4

Ingredients

- 1 sliced medium-sized tomato
- 4 slices of bread
- 8 tablespoons of shredded mozzarella cheese
- 8 tablespoons of diced avocado
- Salt and ground black pepper

Preparation method

Preheat the oven to a temperature of 4000F

Place the bread slices on the baking pan and top each slice with 2 tablespoons of avocado and 2 tablespoons of cheese

Bake for about 10 minutes until the cheese melts and the bread browns

To serve top with the tomatoes, season with pepper and salt

7. Strawberry Buckwheat Porridge

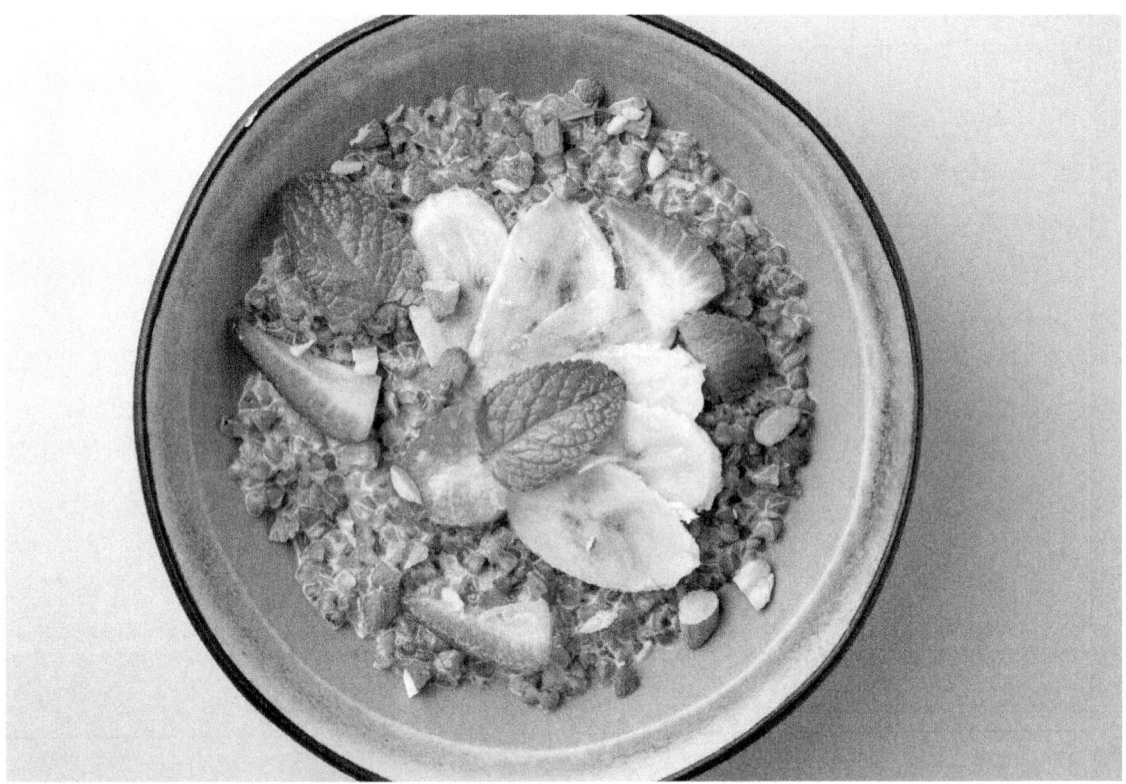

A fantastic and healthy treat to kick off your day. Strawberry buckwheat porridge is not only loaded with calcium, iron, and phosphorous but also a great source of antioxidants and vitamins to boost the immune system. Try out on our simple recipe with a wonderful taste to boost your mood.

Preparation time: 25 minutes **Number of servings:** 2

Ingredients

- 1 cup of chopped strawberries
- ½ cup of buckwheat groats
- 2 teaspoons of honey
- 2 sticks of cinnamon
- 1 cup of unsweetened almond milk
- 2 ½ cups of water
- ¼ teaspoon of salt

Preparation method

Add water and cinnamon into a saucepan and bring it to boil

Stir in the buckwheat and cook on a medium flame for about 15 minutes

Discard the cinnamon, stir in the almond milk and honey

Pour the porridge into two bowls, top each bowl with ½ cup of strawberries and enjoy

8. Oats Veggie Pancake

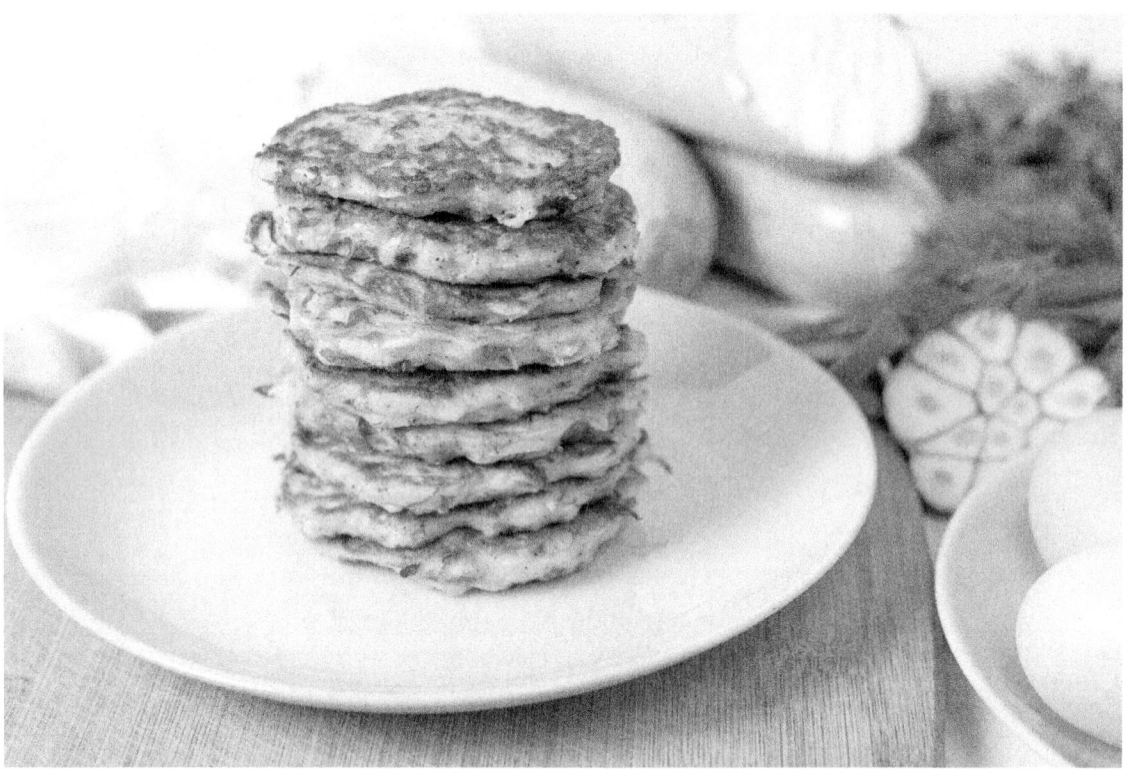

Wondering what to make for breakfast? Prepare this colourful low-calorie vegetable pancake with loads of vitamins to boost the immune system. You can make your oat flour and store it in an airtight container to save your mornings.

Preparation time: 35 minutes **Number of servings:** 7

Ingredients

- 1 cup of oat flour
- ½ cup of finely chopped spinach
- ½ cup of grated carrots
- 2 tablespoons of finely chopped coriander
- 3 ½ teaspoons of olive oil
- 2 teaspoons of chopped green chilies
- 1 cup of water
- Some green chutney

Preparation method

Into a bowl, add in the flour, spinach, carrots, coriander, chilies, water, and combine to make the batter

Place a skillet on medium heat and grease it with ¼ teaspoon of oil

Scoop a spoon full of batter on the skillet and spread it to form a circular disk

Cook both sides until they brown and repeat the procedure with the rest of the batter

Serve with green chutney

9. Spiced Quinoa

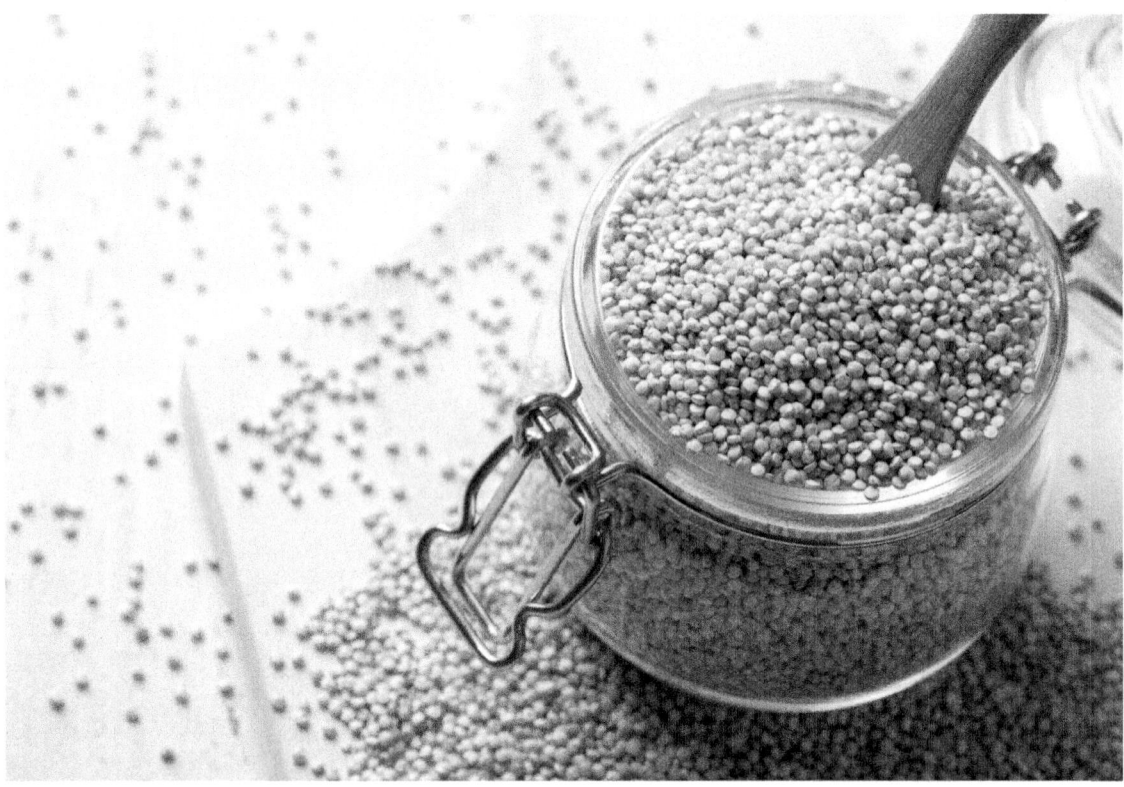

Try out on this healthy breakfast recipe of hot cereal with an intriguing aroma. The blend of spices gives it an amazing taste to satisfy the taste buds.

Preparation time: 35 minutes **Number of servings:** 2

Ingredients

- 1 cup of quinoa
- 1 cup of water
- ½ teaspoon of cinnamon
- 1 cup of low-fat milk
- 2 tablespoons of honey
- ½ teaspoon of vanilla extract
- 1/8 teaspoon of ground nutmeg
- 1/8 teaspoon of ground ginger
- 2 teaspoons of raisins
- ¼ teaspoon of salt
- 1 egg white

Preparation method

Sieve and wash the quinoa with cold water

Heat a saucepan over medium-high heat, add the quinoa and cook-stir for about 4 minutes until fragrant

Stir in the milk, cinnamon, water, ginger, nutmeg, salt and bring to boil

Minimize the heat and simmer uncovered for about 20 minutes until the quinoa is tender

Switch off the heat, stir in the honey and vanilla and set aside

Into a bowl whisk in the egg white, stir in the hot cereal(one tablespoon at a time) until the egg white is fully incorporated

Stir in the raisins and return the mixture into the saucepan

Cook over medium-low heat for about 4 minutes until it thickens

Serve and enjoy

10. Scrambled Egg with Broccoli

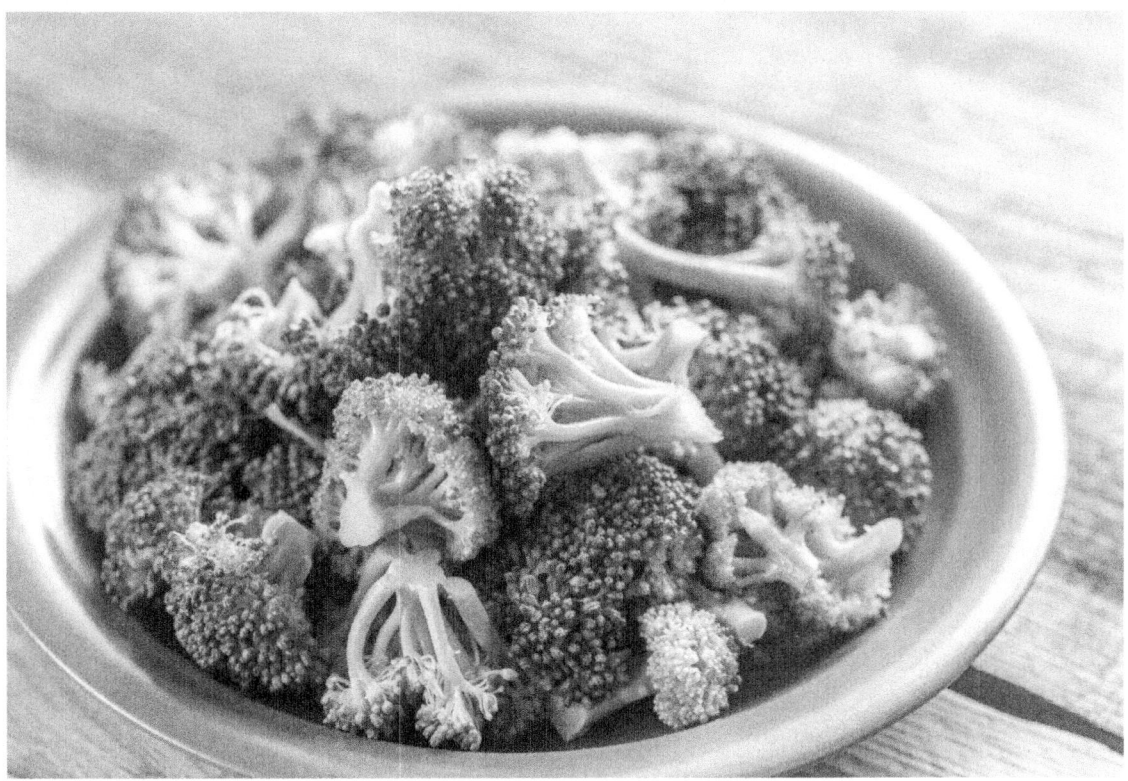

If you are looking for an easy and healthy breakfast fix, try out on our broccoli egg recipe that is packed with fiber, calcium potassium vitamins to keep your body healthy. Create a delicious vegetable filling that you can serve on a toast.

Preparation time: 5 minutes **Number of servings:** 1

Ingredients

- 2 eggs
- 1 teaspoon of water
- 2 teaspoons of olive oil
- ¼ cup of sliced onion
- 1 teaspoon of grated parmesan cheese
- ¼ teaspoon of dried thyme
- ½ cup of chopped broccoli
- 1 slice of whole-wheat toast
- Salt and ground black pepper

Preparation method

Into a bowl, whisk in the eggs, water, cheese, salt and pepper

Heat 2 teaspoons of oil in a pan, sauté the onion and thyme for about 3 minutes

Add the broccoli and cook for more minutes

Add in the egg mixture and scramble until set

Serve over a slice of bread and enjoy

11. Coconut Carrot Porridge

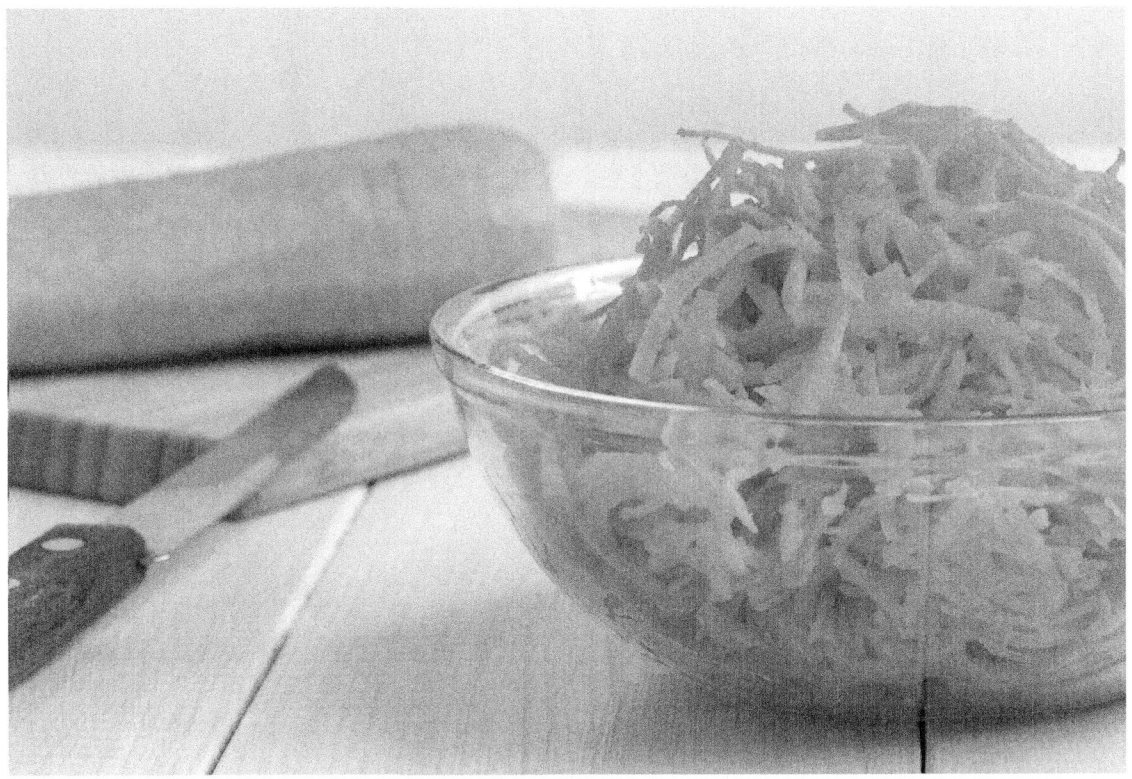

Start the day with this simple and delicious carrot porridge packed with a natural blend of flavours from the herbs. It is ideal for patients with poor appetite. You can use any other plant milk such as almond in place of coconut milk.

Preparation time: 20 minutes Number of servings 4

Ingredients

- 4 carrots, grated
- 2 tablespoons of honey(optional)
- 1 tablespoon of coconut butter
- 7 cups of coconut milk
- 1 1/3 cups of raisins
- 2 ½ cups of porridge oats
- 1 teaspoon of freshly grated nutmeg
- 2 teaspoons of cinnamon

Preparation method

Into a saucepan, add in the butter, carrots, milk, oats, nutmeg, cinnamon, and raisins. Cook-stir for about 15 minutes over medium heat until the carrots and oats are soft

Add some coconut milk to achieve the desired thickness

Serve with honey

Smoothies

12. Blueberry Orange Smoothie with Muffin

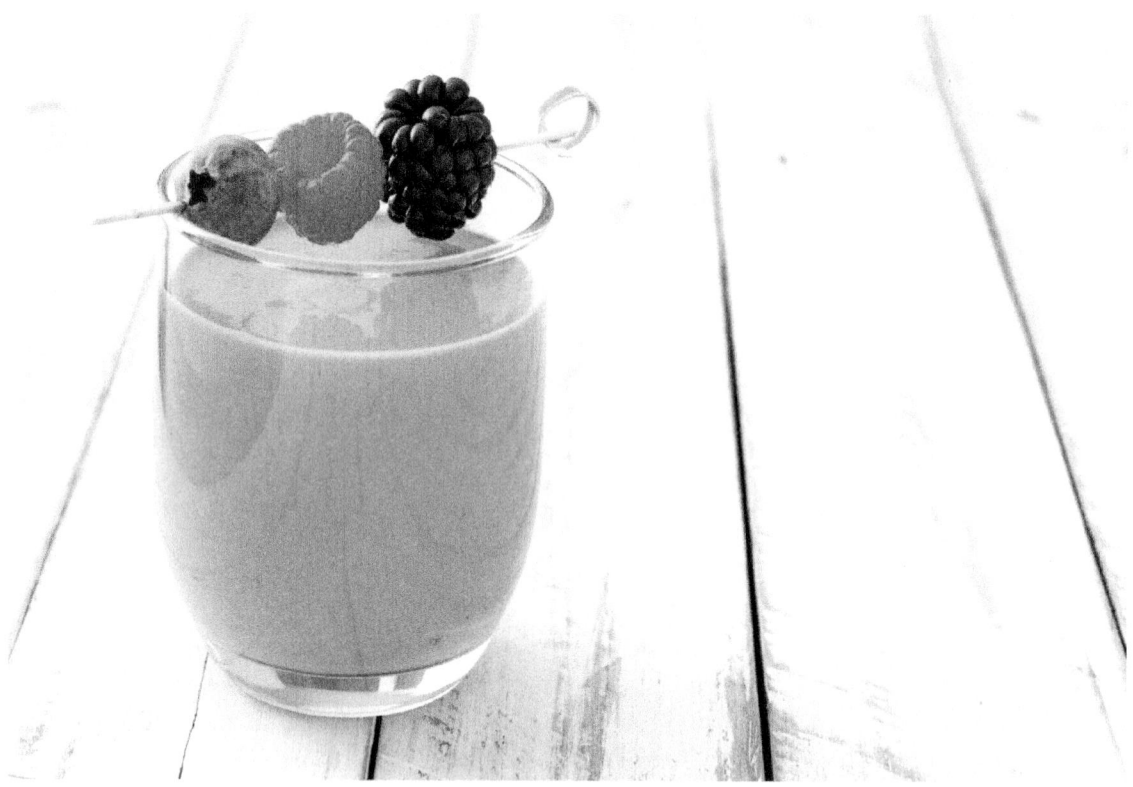

If you are looking for a fast and convenient way to consume many nutrients, then the blueberry orange smoothie recipe is an ideal choice. This delicious smoothie will help infighting off nausea and keep you feeling full for long.

Preparation time: 5 minutes **Number of servings:** 1

Ingredients

- ½ cup of orange segments
- ½ cup of frozen blueberries
- ½ cup of almond milk
- 1 teaspoon of vanilla extract
- ½ of frozen banana
- 1 toasted English muffin
- 1 tablespoon of peanut butter

Preparation method

Into a blender, add in the oranges, blueberries, banana, vanilla and almond milk

Blend until smooth and pour the mixture into a glass

Spread the toast with butter and enjoy

13. Avocado Broccoli Smoothie

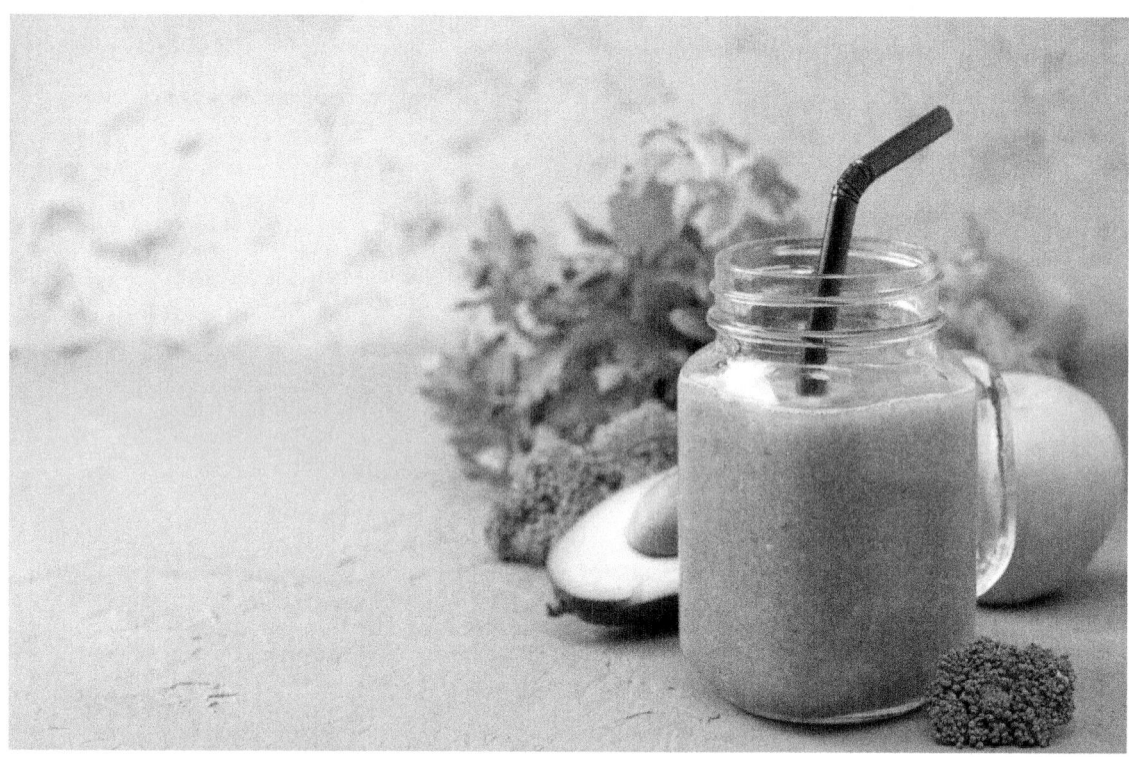

Try out on this flavorful smoothie that is an ideal breakfast for children with low appetite due to the cancer medication. This gluten-free smoothie is rich in healthy fat, fiber, and antioxidants to help in fighting cancerous cells.

Preparation time: 5 minutes **Number of servings:** 4

Ingredients

- 1 medium-sized banana
- 1 cup of broccoli
- 1 cup of cherries
- 1 teaspoon of ground flaxseed
- 1 cup of pomegranate juice
- 1 medium-sized avocado

Preparation method

Into a blender, add in the banana, broccoli, cherries, flaxseeds, pomegranate juice, avocado

Blend until smooth and serve

14. Watermelon Smoothie

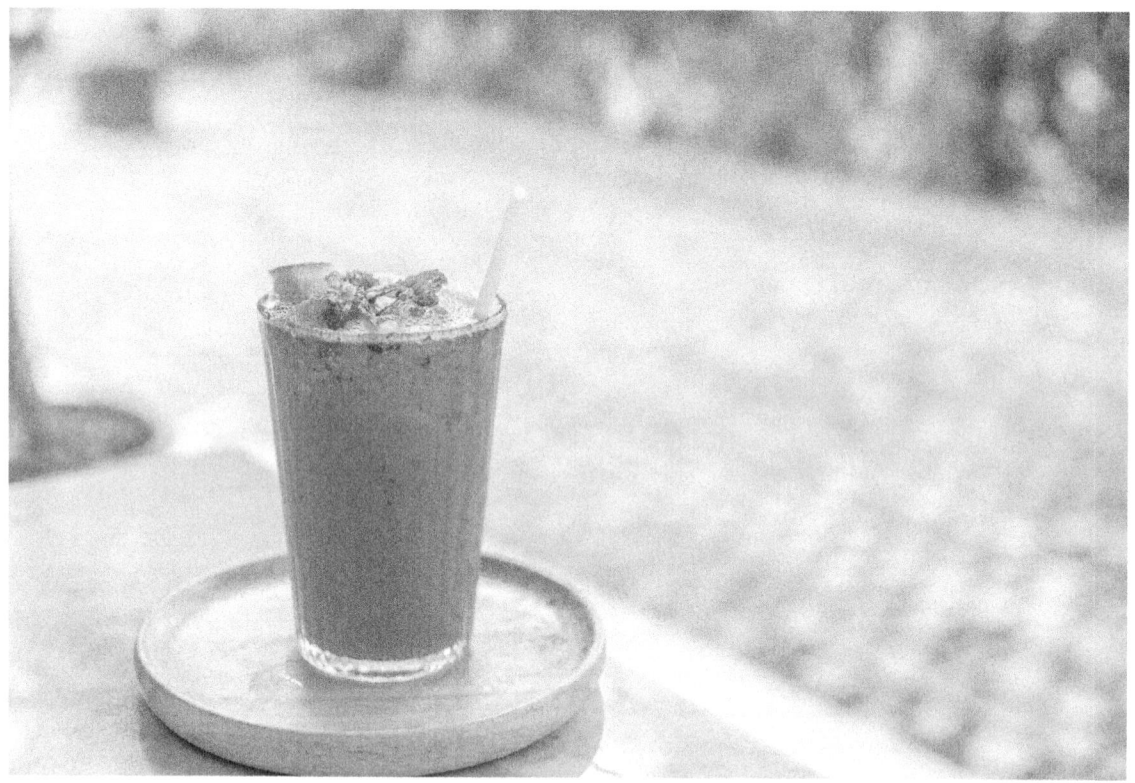

Create a delicious summertime smoothie from fresh herbs, cucumber, and watermelon to relieve nausea and other digestive issues. Although it is low in calories is keeps the body hydrated.

Preparation time: 5 minutes **Number of servings:** 2

Ingredients

- 2 cups of chopped watermelon
- ½ cucumber
- 2 sprigs of mint
- Honey to taste(optional)

Preparation method

Into a blender, add in the watermelon, cucumber, and mint

Blend until smooth and then add some honey to taste

Serve and enjoy

15. Ginger Carrot Beet Smoothie

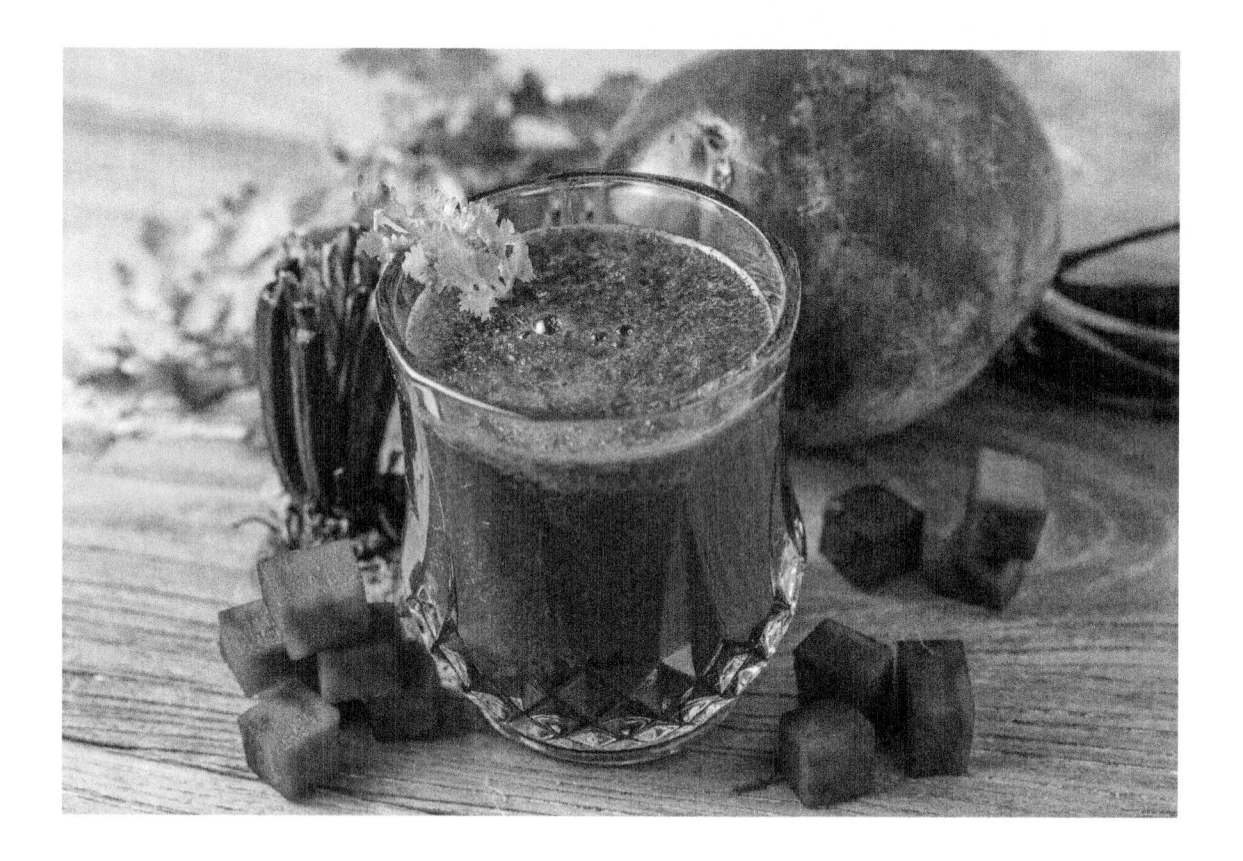

A perfect breakfast for cancer patients with low appetite. This smoothie is not only delicious and flavorful, but the best nutrient-packed drink. It has a delightful colour and nutrients to keep someone fueled for the day.

Preparation time: 5 minutes **Number of servings:** 2

Ingredients

- 2 peeled and diced medium-sized beetroots
- 2 peeled red apples
- 3 medium-sized carrots, peeled and diced
- A piece of ginger root, 2 inches long
- 5 stalks of celery
- A handful of cilantro

Preparation method

Into a blender, add in the beetroots, apples, carrots, celery, ginger and cilantro

Blend until smooth and serve

Soups

16. Scallion Asparagus Soup

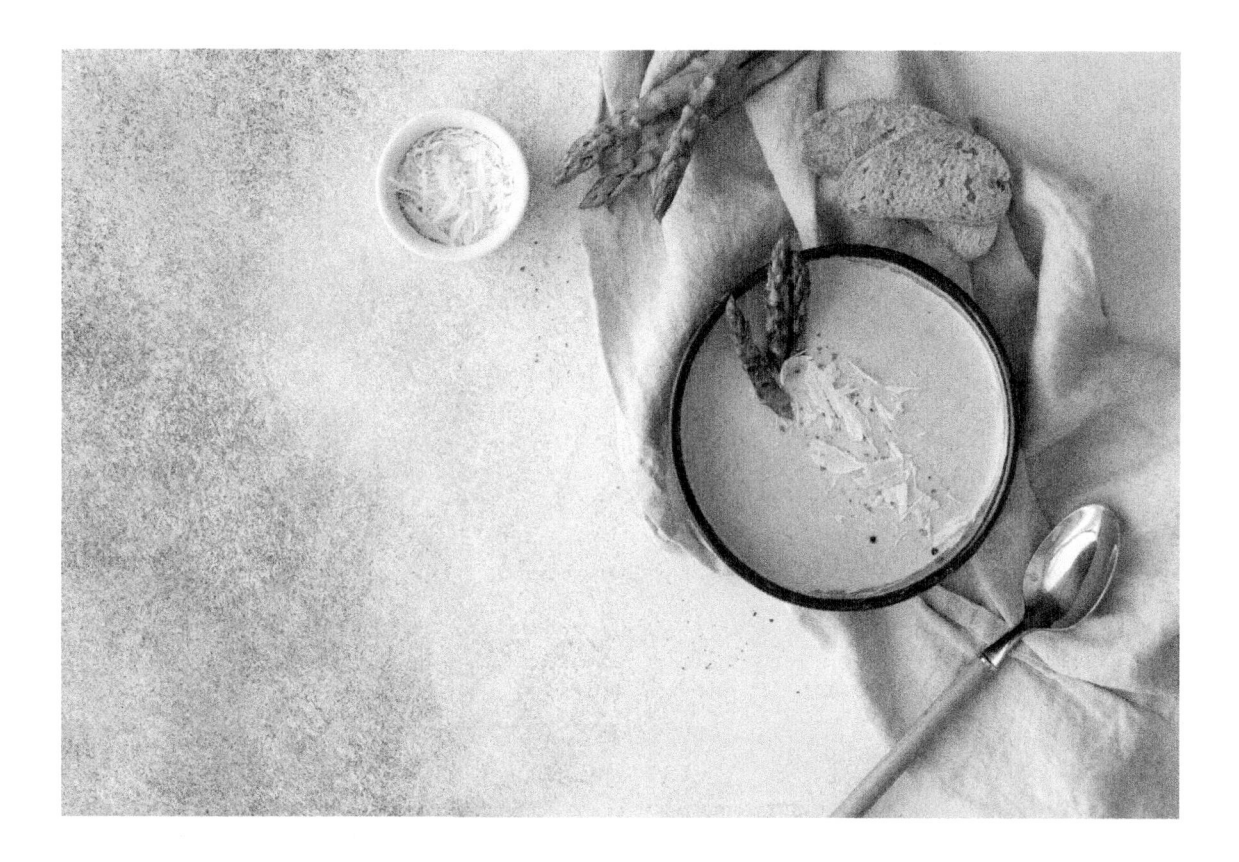

If the patient does not feel like chewing on anything, then try out on Scallion Asparagus soup that is not only flavorful but also nutritious. You can adapt the recipe and slash out the scallions to suit patients on a low microbial diet. The skimmed milk gives a creamy touch to the soup.

Preparation time: 30 minutes **Number of servings:** 6

Ingredients

- 1 tablespoon of olive oil
- ½ teaspoon of dried thyme
- ¼ cup of sliced almonds
- 1 cup of skimmed milk
- 1 ½ lb. of asparagus with ends trimmed
- 6 thinly sliced scallions
- 28 oz of fat-free, low sodium chicken broth
- 2 thinly sliced leeks
- 15 oz of white beans, rinsed and drained
- 1 tablespoon of low-sodium soy sauce
- Salt and white pepper

Preparation method

1. Over medium heat, roast the nuts in a pan for about 6 minutes until golden, (occasionally swirl the nuts to avoid burning). Set them aside

Over medium heat, heat the oil in a saucepan, add the and four sliced scallions, cook-stir for about 5 minutes, add the chicken broth, salt, white pepper thyme and bring to boil

Add the beans and asparagus, bring to boil and simmer covered for about 12 minutes until the vegetables are soft

In a blender, puree the soup until smooth

Add the puree back into the saucepan to cook over medium heat, stir in the milk and cook for about 3 minutes

Serve into bowls and garnish with the almonds and the scallions

17. Onion Butternut Squash Soup

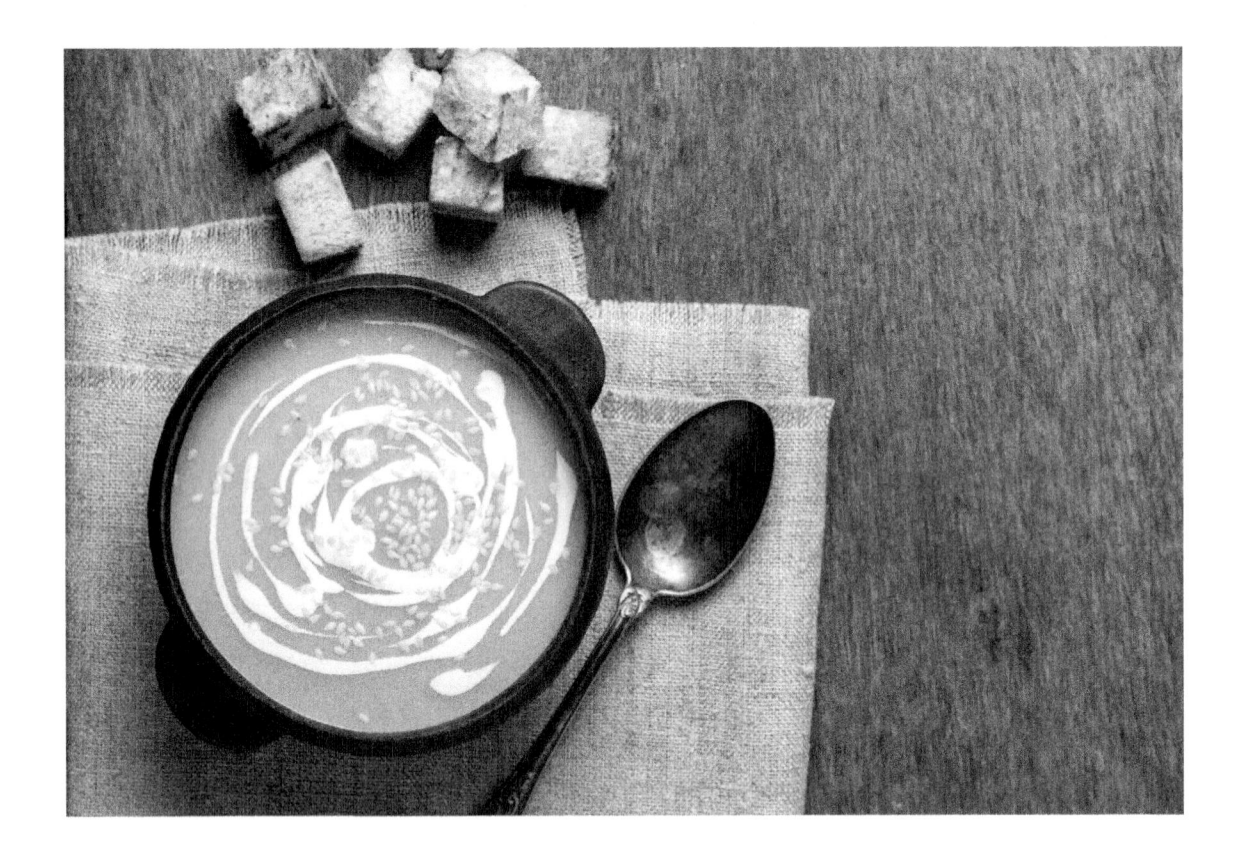

An ideal treat for patients with low appetite. This orange soup comes with a natural sweetness besides numerous health benefits to the body. Onion butternut squash soup is packed with beta-carotene that aids in converting needed vitamin A to boost the immune system.

Preparation time: 30 minutes **Number of servings:** 6

Ingredients

- 2 small apples, peeled and sliced
- 1 pound of thinly sliced red onions
- ¼ cup of maple syrup
- 1 ½ tablespoons of canola oil
- 2 pounds of squash, peeled and diced
- 4 cups of chicken broth, low sodium

Preparation method

Over medium heat, heat the oil in a saucepan, and sauté the onions until they are just brown, add in the apples and cook for about 3 minutes

Stir in the squash, add the broth and bring to boil

Simmer while covered until the vegetables are tender and cooked through

Cool slightly and puree the soup in a food processor until smooth

Stir in the maple syrup and then serve

18. Apple Carrot Soup

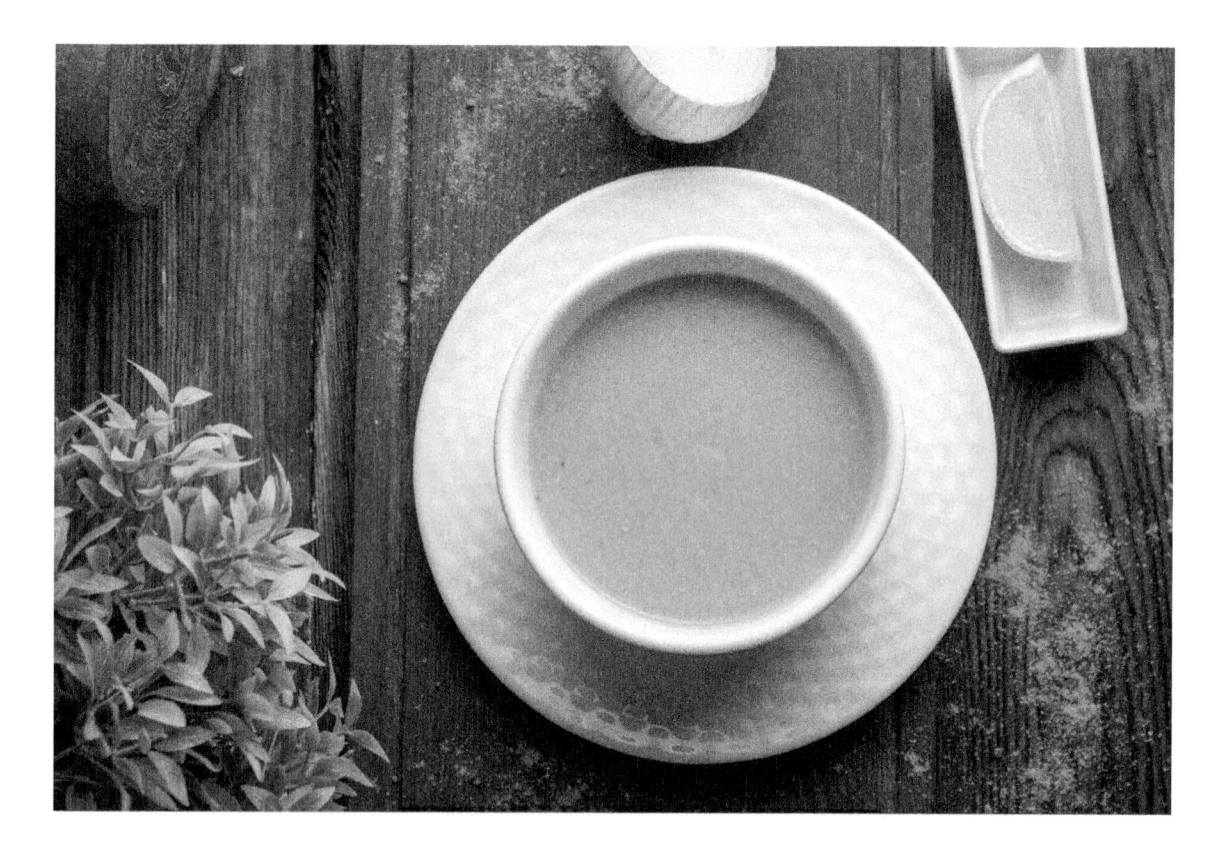

A perfect soup to boost your immunity and ward off infections. The soup is not only filling but also rich in fiber to soothe the stomach. You can prepare it in advance and refrigerate it to save time.

Preparation time: 40 minutes **Number of servings:** 4

Ingredients

- 1 medium-sized chopped onion
- 1 medium-sized chopped leek
- 1 apple, peeled, cored and chopped
- 3 cups of low sodium chicken broth
- 1 tablespoon of canola oil
- 1 pound of chopped carrots
- Salt and ground black pepper

Preparation method

Over medium-high heat, heat oil in a saucepan and sauté the onions and leek until soft for about 4 minutes

Add in the carrots and apple, cover the saucepan, minimize the heat and cook for about 10 minutes

Add in the broth, cover and cook for about 20 minutes until the carrots are soft

Allow cooling and puree the mixture using a food processor

Season with pepper and salt

Serve and enjoy

19. Red Lentil Soup

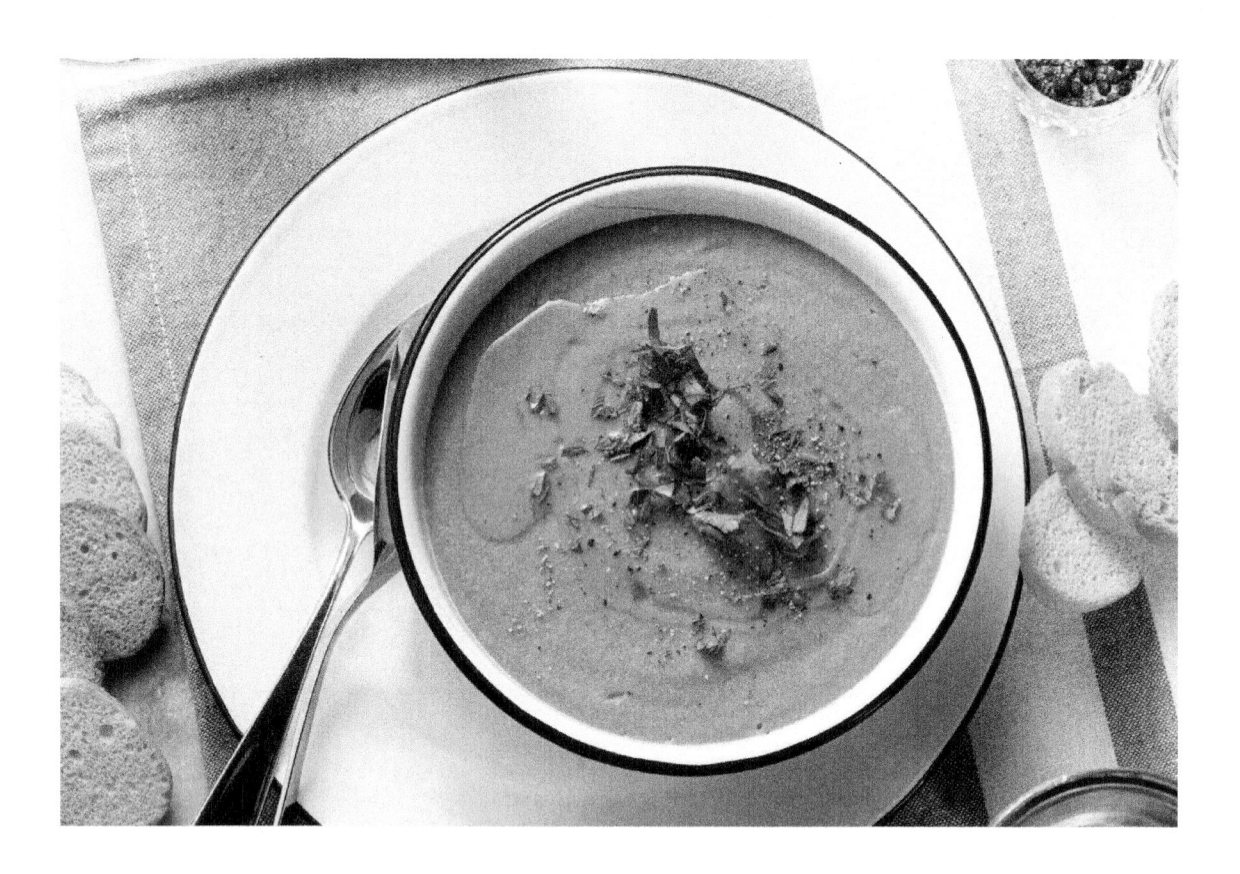

Try out on this delicious and filling veggie soup and enjoy its nutritional benefits. Red lentil soup is an excellent source of potassium, niacin, iron, and foliate. It is not only easy to make but also good for patients with low appetite.

Preparation time: 40 minutes **Number of servings:** 4

Ingredients

- 1 tablespoon of unsalted butter
- 1 medium-sized chopped onion
- Salt
- 1 cup of lentils
- 0.5 pounds of diced tomatoes
- ¼ teaspoon of chili powder
- ¼ teaspoon of ground coriander
- ½ teaspoon of ground cumin
- 2 garlic cloves, thinly sliced
- 2 finely chopped celery ribs
- 1 finely chopped carrot
- 4 cups of water

Preparation method

Over medium heat, melt the butter in a saucepan, add in the onion, garlic, celery, carrots, and cook until soft for about 5 minutes

Stir in the cumin, chili and coriander, cook for about 3 minutes until fragrant

Stir in the tomatoes and cook for about 2 minutes

Add in the lentils and water, season with salt, cover and simmer for about 30 minutes

Allow cooling and puree with a blender or food processor

Serve and enjoy

20. Pea Vegetable Soup

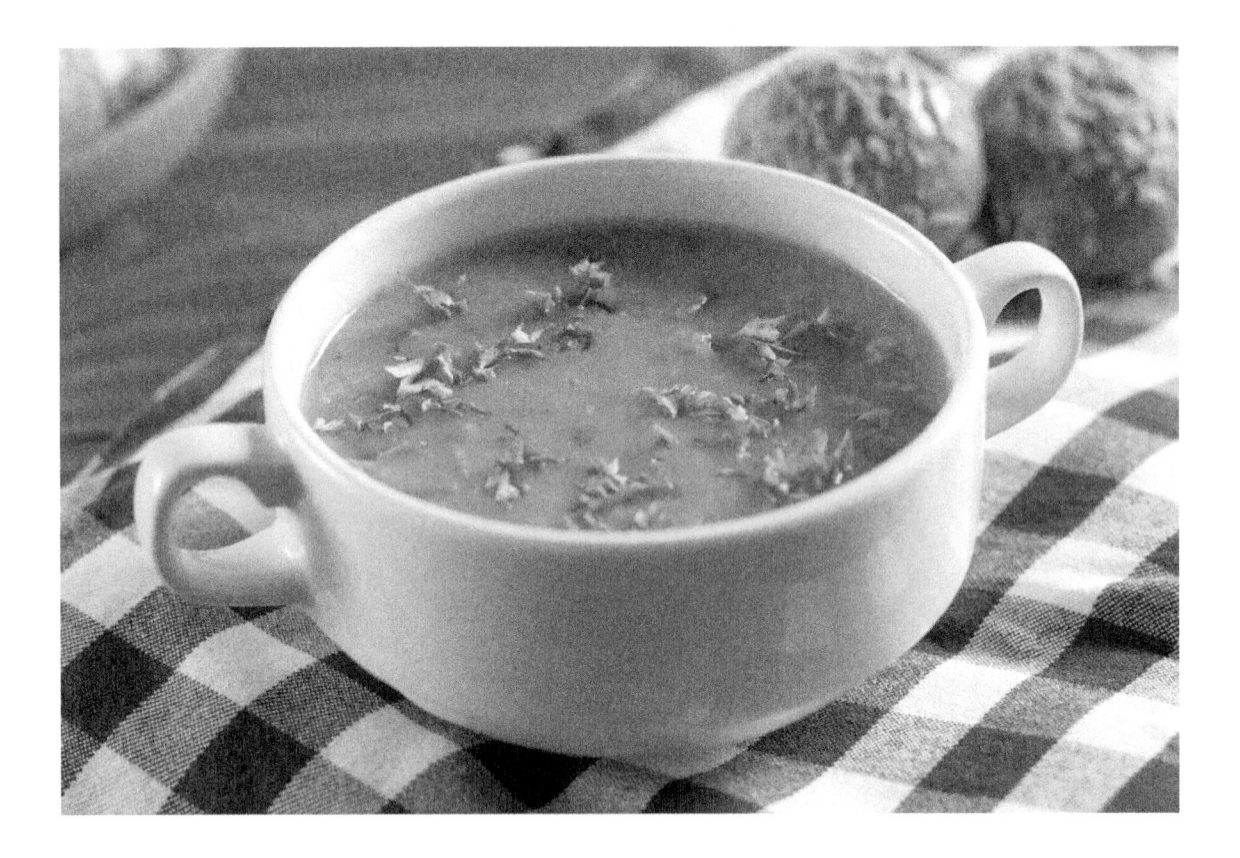

Boost your immune system with our delicious and yet simple to make vegetable soup. This nutritious soup comes with loads of vitamin A, C, and folate. It is suitable for patients with feeding problems because it contains fiber that aids in digestion.

Preparation time: 35 minutes **Number of servings:** 4

Ingredients

- 1 medium-sized onion, chopped
- 1 tablespoon of butter
- 1 medium-sized peeled and diced sweet potato
- 1 white potato, peeled and diced
- 3 cups of chicken broth
- ½ cup of green beans
- 1/8 teaspoon of paprika
- 1 large carrot, peeled and diced
- 1 zucchini, thinly sliced
- ½ cup of green peas
- 1 cup of broccoli florets, chopped
- Salt and pepper

Preparation method

Over medium heat, heat the butter in a saucepan and sauté the onions, stir in the carrots, potatoes, beans, zucchini and cook for a minute

Add the broth and bring to a boil, cover and simmer for about 30 minutes

Add in the peas, paprika, broccoli and cook for about 10 minutes

Season with pepper and salt

Puree and serve

Main course meals

21. Cauliflower, Broccoli and Tofu

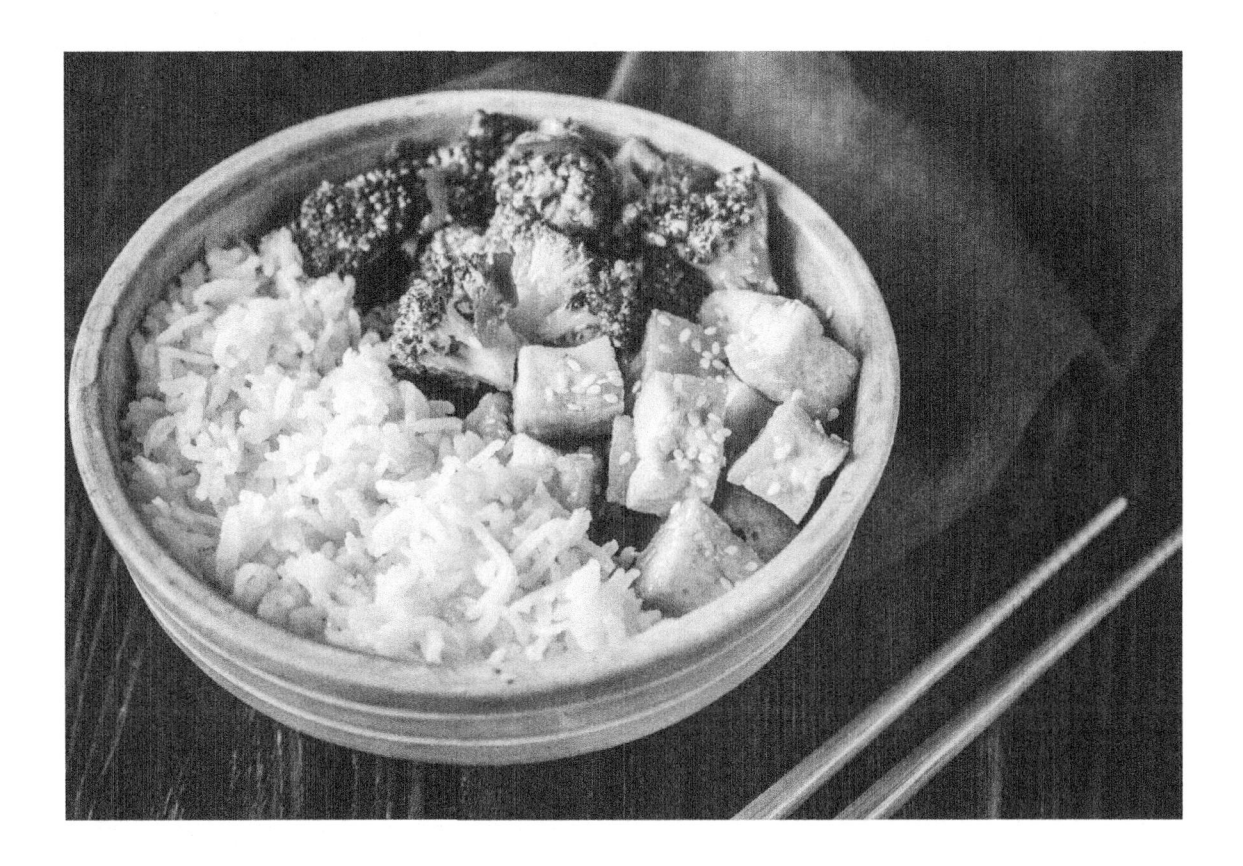

Try out on our hearty tofu meal that is filled with proteins, vitamins, and minerals with numerous health benefits. Tofu blends on well with the spiced vegetables to satisfy the taste buds of the patient.

Preparation time: 20 minutes **Number of servings:** 4

Ingredients

- 1 teaspoon of ground coriander
- 1 teaspoon of ground cumin
- 2 tablespoons of canola oil
- 1 teaspoon of grated ginger
- 1 small onion, cut into wedges
- 1 ½ cups of broccoli florets
- 2 minced garlic cloves
- 12 oz of tofu, cut into small pieces
- 1 cup of cauliflower florets
- ½ teaspoon of chili powder

Preparation method

Over medium-high heat, heat a skillet until hot, add in the coriander, cumin, and cook-stir for a minute

Gently add in the oil, chili and garlic and stir for about 2 minutes

Stir in the onions and cook for 2 more minutes until soft

Add in the broccoli and cauliflower and cook until crispy

Toss in the tofu to warm through and coat with spices

Serve and enjoy

22. Black Beans Vegetable Casserole

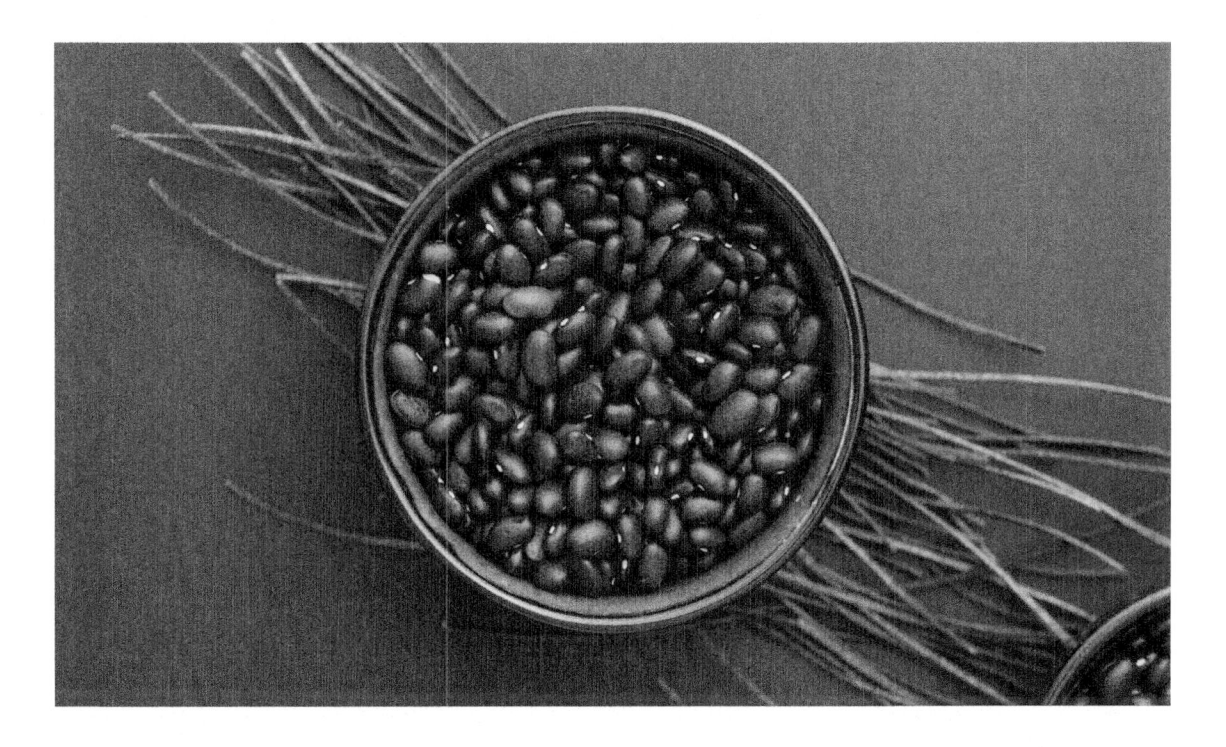

Try out on our bean recipe with an outstanding amount of antioxidants and fiber that reduce the risk of cancer by protecting colon cells. This delicious meal is easy to prepare, and it is ideal for patients on a low microbial diet.

Preparation time: 1 hour **Number of servings:** 8

Ingredients

- 1 chopped large onion
- 1 green capsicum, chopped
- 2 minced garlic cloves
- 1 tablespoon of canola oil
- ½ teaspoon of ground cumin
- 1 tablespoon of chili powder
- 14 oz of drained and rinsed black beans
- 14 oz of drained and rinsed pinto beans
- 28 oz of pureed tomatoes
- 12 corn tortillas
- 16 oz of frozen corn, thawed
- ¼ teaspoon of hot sauce (optional)
- 1 cup of grated low fat jack cheese
- Salt and ground black pepper

Preparation method

Preheat the oven to a temperature of 3500F

Over medium heat, heat oil in a saucepan and sauté the capsicum, garlic and onion for about 5 minutes until soft

Add in the beans, tomatoes, corn, chili, hot sauce, cumin, salt and pepper, Minimize the heat and simmer for about 15 minutes

Place 1/3 of the bean mixture in a 9x13-inch baking dish, layer six tortillas on top, place the ½ of remaining bean mixture on top, layer with the remaining tortillas and top with the other ½ of the bean mixture

Sprinkle the cheese on the bean mixture and bake for about 40 minutes until hot and bubbly

Allow cooling and serve

23. Lamb Cutlets with Mashed Potatoes, Garlic and Peas

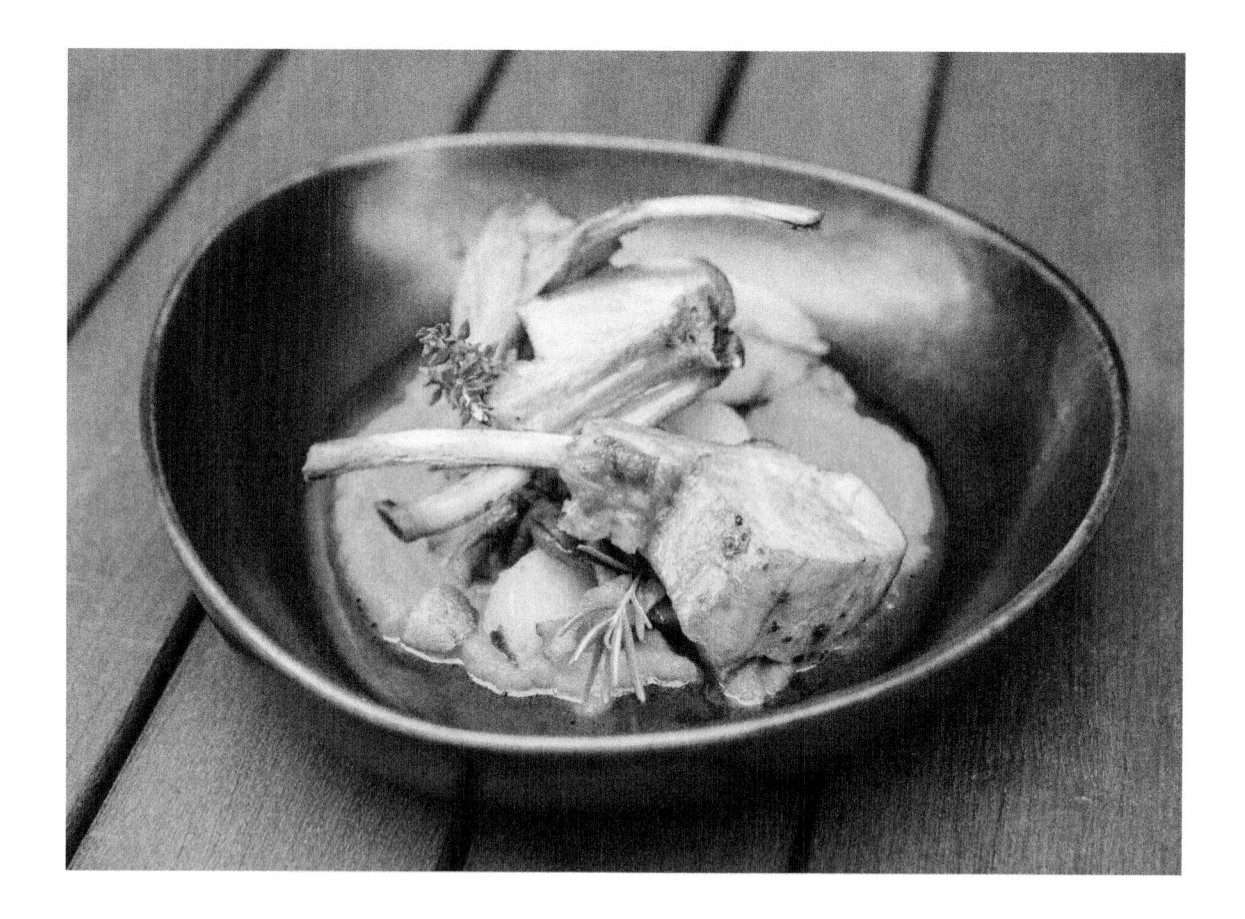

A gorgeous meal to prepare for a cancer patient. It comes with an amazing flavour and taste that will awaken their taste buds. This easy to prepare dinner is packed with proteins and vitamins that lower the risk of cancer.

Preparation time: 1 hour **Number of servings:** 4

Ingredients

- 4 white potatoes, peeled and cubed
- 4, 1 ¼ inch thick slices of lamb steak
- ½ cup of milk
- 2 tablespoons of olive oil
- 2 cups of frozen peas, thawed
- 2 tablespoons of butter
- Salt and black pepper
- 4 minced garlic cloves
- ½ cup of chicken broth
- ½ cup of white wine
- 2 tablespoons of lemon juice
- ½ cup of crème Fraiche
- ¼ cup of finely chopped chives
- A handful of finely chopped mint
- A handful of finely chopped parsley

Preparation method

Boil the potatoes in water over medium-high heat until soft for about 15 minutes and set aside

Meanwhile, season the lamb with salt and pepper

Heat oil in a skillet over medium-high heat, cook the meat until it browns on both sides for about 8 minutes

Minimize the heat and stir in the butter, ½ of the garlic, and cook for 2 more minutes

Add in the white wine, simmer until the wire reduces by almost half for about 3 minutes

Add in a splash of chicken broth and allow it to bubble up, stir in the lemon juice and set aside

Drain the potatoes, add the remaining broth, crème Fraiche ¼ cup of milk, parsley, mint, remaining garlic, peas and seasoning

Mash the mixture and add the milk to achieve the desired thickness

Serve with the lamb and enjoy

24. Lentil Dhal with Rice

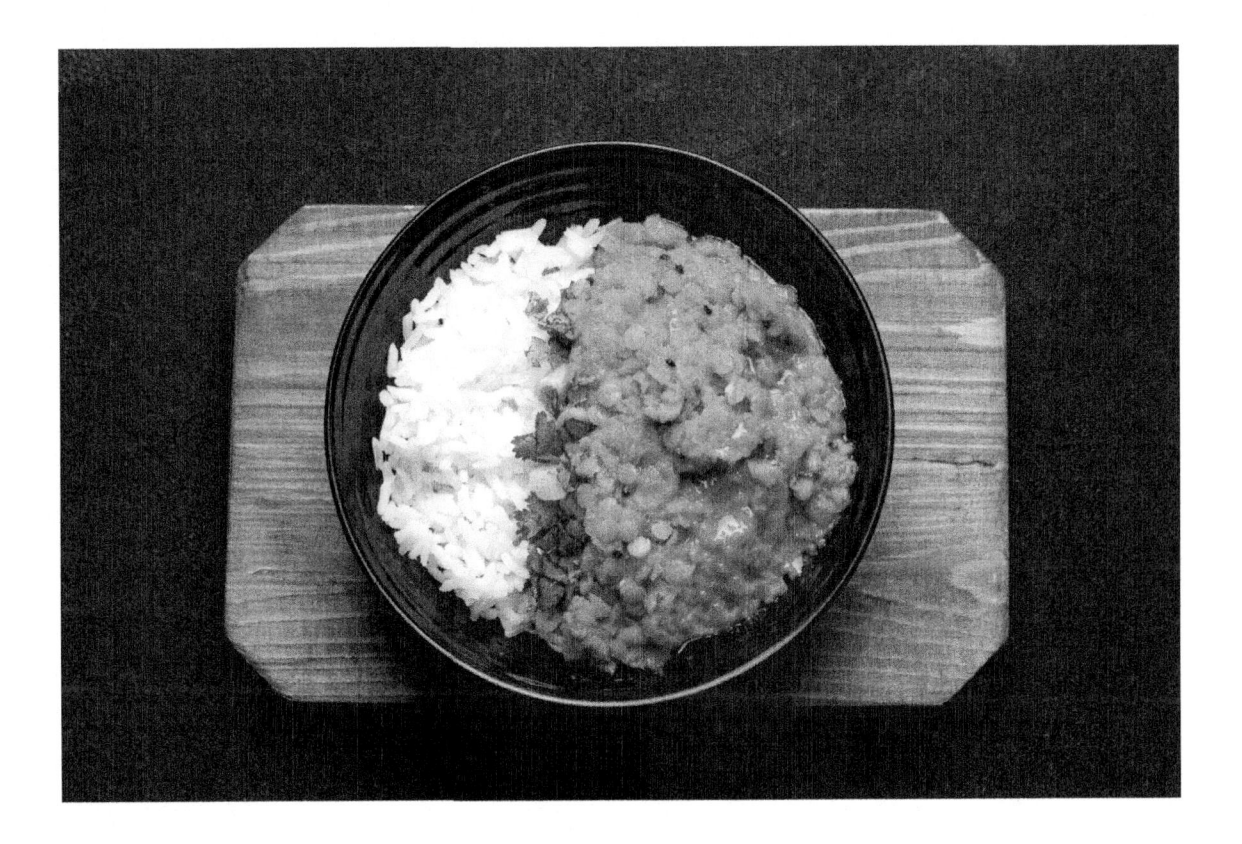

A perfect meal for a vegetarian patient that is full of antioxidants to fight bacteria. You can adjust the amount of chili for a mild taste or skip it. Besides, you can also replace the ghee with a light oil such as grape seed oil and the results will be amazing.

Preparation time: 30 minutes **Number of servings:** 4

Ingredients

- 1 ½ teaspoons of ground turmeric
- 14 oz of red lentils
- 4 ½ cups of vegetable broth
- 1 tablespoon of ghee
- 1 teaspoon of mustard seeds
- 1 teaspoon of cumin seeds
- 1 teaspoon of chili flakes
- 1 peeled and sliced onion
- 2 minced garlic cloves
- Salt
- A handful of roughly chopped coriander

Preparation method

Over medium-high heat, add the lentils, broth, turmeric, and some salt in a saucepan and bring to a boil

Simmer for about 25 minutes and occasionally stir to avoid the sticking

Meanwhile, heat a smaller saucepan until hot and melt in the ghee, add in the cumin seeds, mustard seeds and cover until the seeds start to pop up.

Uncover when the popping stops and add in the onions, chili, garlic and fry for few minutes until the onions are soft

Stir in the spice mixture to the lentils and garnish with coriander

Serve with boiled rice.

25. Noodles with Ginger and Peanut Sauce

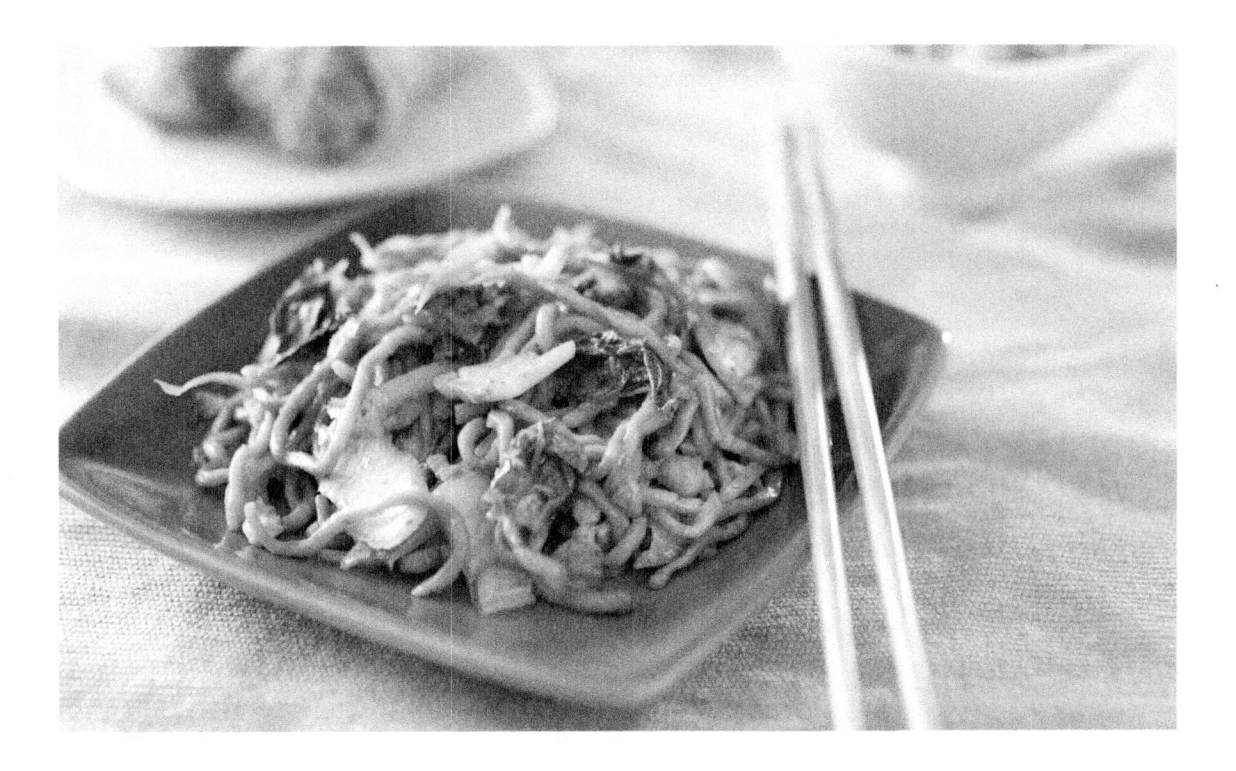

This recipe will impress all the noodle lovers. The colour blend of the vegetables and the ginger flavour will awaken the taste buds of the patient. It is an ideal dish for patients on a low microbial diet.

Preparation time: 30 minutes **Number of servings:** 4

Ingredients

- 1 pack of whole-grain Udon noodles
- 1 large, sliced carrot
- 2 tablespoons of sesame oil
- 1 broccoli head cut into smaller pieces
- 3 red onions, finely chopped
- ½ cup of warm water
- 1 tablespoon of low-sodium soy sauce
- ¼ teaspoon of cayenne pepper (optional)
- 1/3 cup of peanut butter
- 2 tablespoons grated ginger root

Preparation method

Cook the udon noodles in boiling water as per the packaging instructions, drain and set aside

Over medium-high heat, heat the oil in a pan, add in the carrots, broccoli, onions and fry for about 5 minutes until lightly cooked

Reduce the heat to low, stir in the noodles for few minutes

To make the dressing, combine the water, soy sauce, ginger, butter and cayenne

Add the dressing in the noodles and stir-fry for a few minutes

Serve and enjoy

26. Salmon with Faro and Caponata

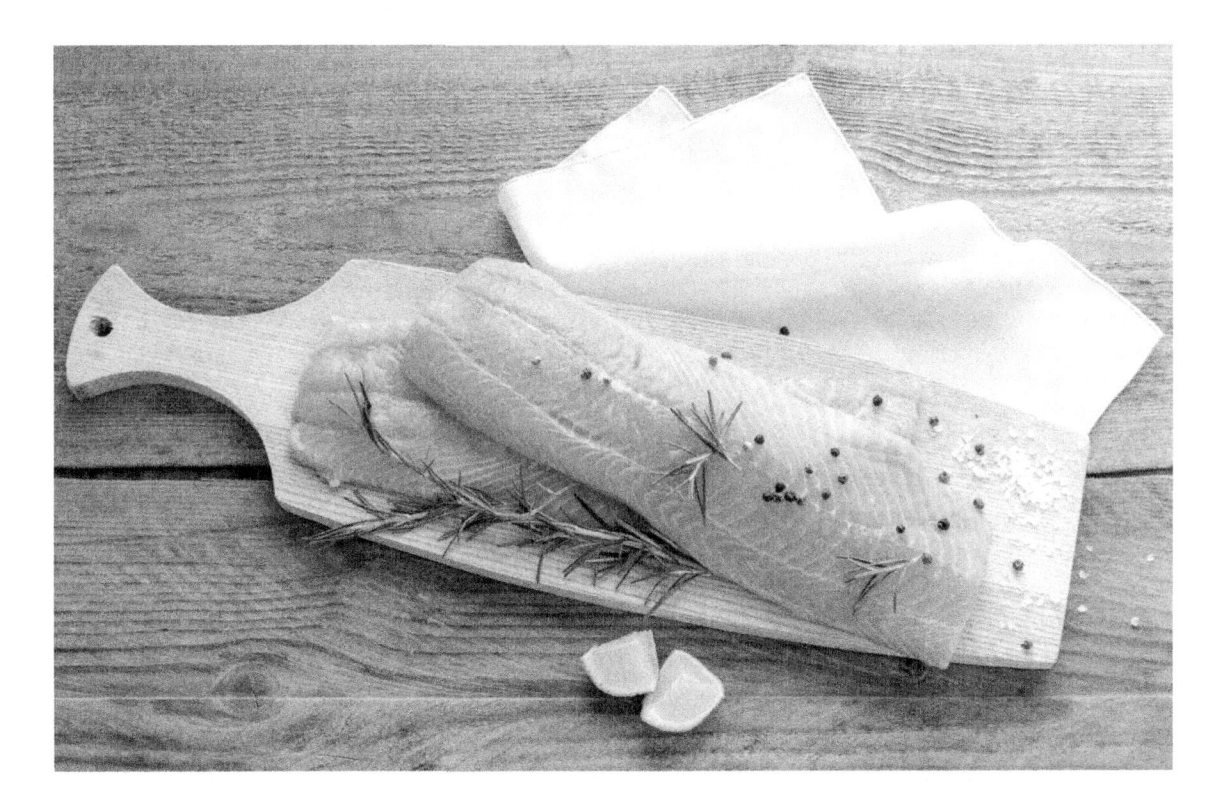

Try out on this simple yet delicious Mediterranean recipe for dinner packed with vegetables and benefit from its nutritional value. It has loads of vitamins and minerals to boost your immune system. You can serve the dish with brown rice though you can swap the vegetables and whole-grain with your favourite.

Preparation time: 50 minutes **Number of servings:** 4

Ingredients

- 2/3 cup of farro
- 2 cups of water
- 1 eggplant diced into 1-inch pieces
- 1 red capsicum, chopped
- 2 tablespoons of rinsed and chopped capers
- 1 summer squash, diced
- 1 small, sliced onion
- 1 ½ cups of cherry tomatoes
- 3 tablespoons of olive oil
- Salt and ground black pepper
- 1 tablespoon of red wine vinegar
- 2 tablespoons of honey
- 1 ¼ pound of wild salmon cut into four
- ½ teaspoon of Italian seasoning
- 4 lemon wedges

Preparation method

Place the racks on the upper and lower thirds of the oven and preheat the oven to a temperature of 4500F and line 2 baking sheet with foil and coat with cooking spray

Into a saucepan, add faro in water and bring to boil, minimize the heat, cover, and simmer for about 30 minutes until just tender. If necessary drain

Into a bowl, add in the capsicum, eggplant, onion, squash, tomatoes, ½ teaspoon of salt, ½ teaspoon of black pepper, oil and toss well

Divide the vegetables between the baking sheets and place them on the racks. Roast for about 25 minutes and stir once at 12 minutes

Return the vegetables in the bowl, stir in the capers honey and vinegar

Into another bowl, season the salmon with Italian seasoning, lemon zest, ½ teaspoon of salt, ½ teaspoon of black pepper

Place them on the baking sheet and roast for about 10 minutes until they are cooked through

Serve the salmon with vegetable caponata, lemon wedges and farro

27. Chicken with green veggies

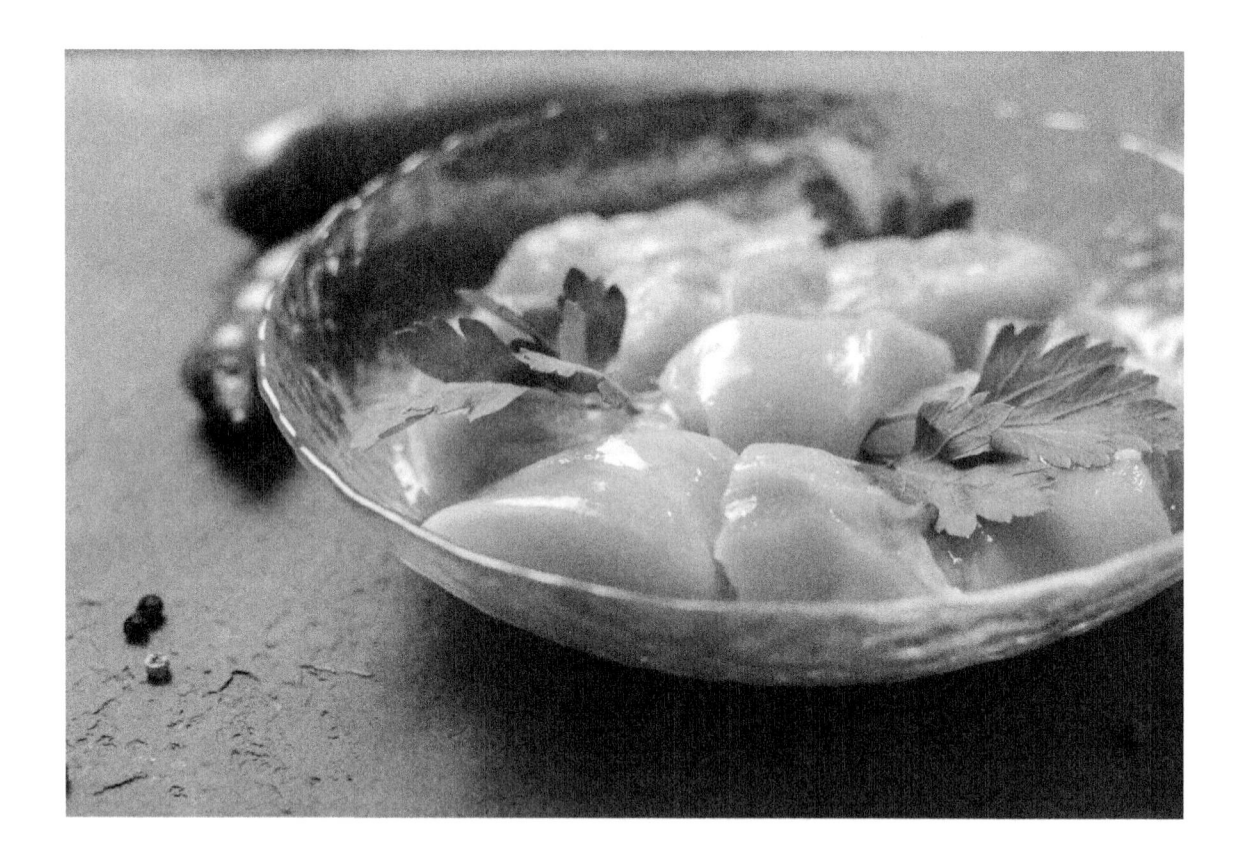

An amazing way to sneak in vegetables to your dinner. Try out on this healthy meal that you can prepare within 30 minutes. The chicken veggie is packed with flavour and nutrients to improve on the immune system.

Preparation time: 30 minutes **Number of servings:** 4

Ingredients

- ¼ cup of lemon juice
- ½ cup of cold water
- ¼ cup of tahini
- ¼ teaspoon of ground cumin
- ½ teaspoon of ground garlic
- 2 cloves of garlic. thinly sliced
- salt
- 1 cup of green beans, trimmed and cut into half
- 1 cup of broccoli florets
- 4 , 4oz chicken cutlets, trimmed
- 2 cups of cooked brown rice
- ¼ cup of chopped cilantro
- 4 cups of thinly chopped kale
- 1 medium-sized red onion
- 2 tablespoons of olive oil
- ¼ teaspoon of ground black pepper

Preparation method

Into a bowl, whisk in the tahini and ¼ cup of water until smooth

Whisk in the minced garlic, lemon juice, ¼ teaspoon of salt, cumin and set aside

Season the chicken with pepper and salt

Over medium heat, heat 1 tablespoon of oil in a skillet and cook the chicken for about 5 minutes on each side

Place the meat on a cutting board and wrap it with foil

Add 1 tablespoon of oil in a clean skillet, sauté the onions for about 2 minutes, cook-stir the sliced garlic for about 30 seconds, add in the broccoli, beans, and cook for 2 minutes

Stir in the kale and 2 tablespoons of water, cover and cook the vegetables for 2 minutes until they are tender and just crispy

Slice the chicken

To serve, divide the rice and vegetables into 4 platters, top with a sliced chicken drizzle with reserved dressing and then sprinkle with the cilantro

28. Chicken with Roast Sweet Potatoes

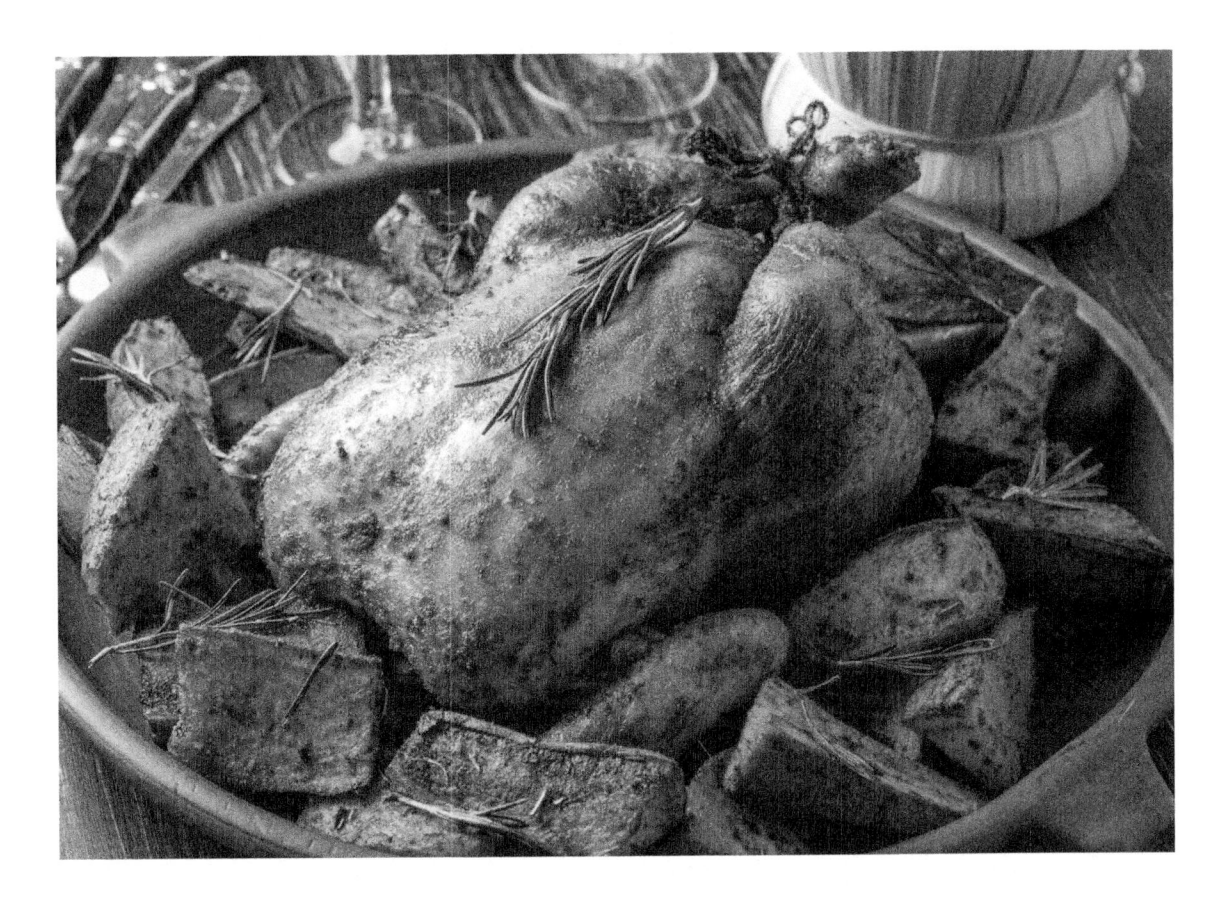

Awaken your appetite with this quick-to-prepare dinner chicken recipe with caramelized sweet potatoes. The meal blends well when served alongside mixed green salad and slices of apple and cheese.

Preparation time: 35 minutes **Number of servings:** 4

Ingredients

- 2 teaspoons of Dijon mustard
- 2 teaspoons of dried thyme
- 2 pound of skinless chicken thigh
- Salt and ground black pepper
- 2 tablespoons of olive oil
- 1 large onion, cut into wedges
- 2 medium-sized peeled and diced sweet potatoes

Preparation method

Place the rack in the lower third of the oven, Preheat the oven to a temperature of 4500F and place a rimmed baking sheet to preheat

Into a bowl, combine the thyme, mustard, 1 tablespoon of olive oil, ¼ teaspoon of pepper, and ¼ teaspoon of salt

Into another bowl, add in the potatoes, onions, 1 tablespoon of oil, ¼ teaspoon of salt, ¼ teaspoon of pepper and toss well to coat

Spread the vegetables in the baking sheet, top with chicken and roast for about 30 minutes or until the thermometer reading inserted on the thigh is 1650F. (stir once at 15 minutes)

Allow cooling and serve

29. Chorizo with pea soup

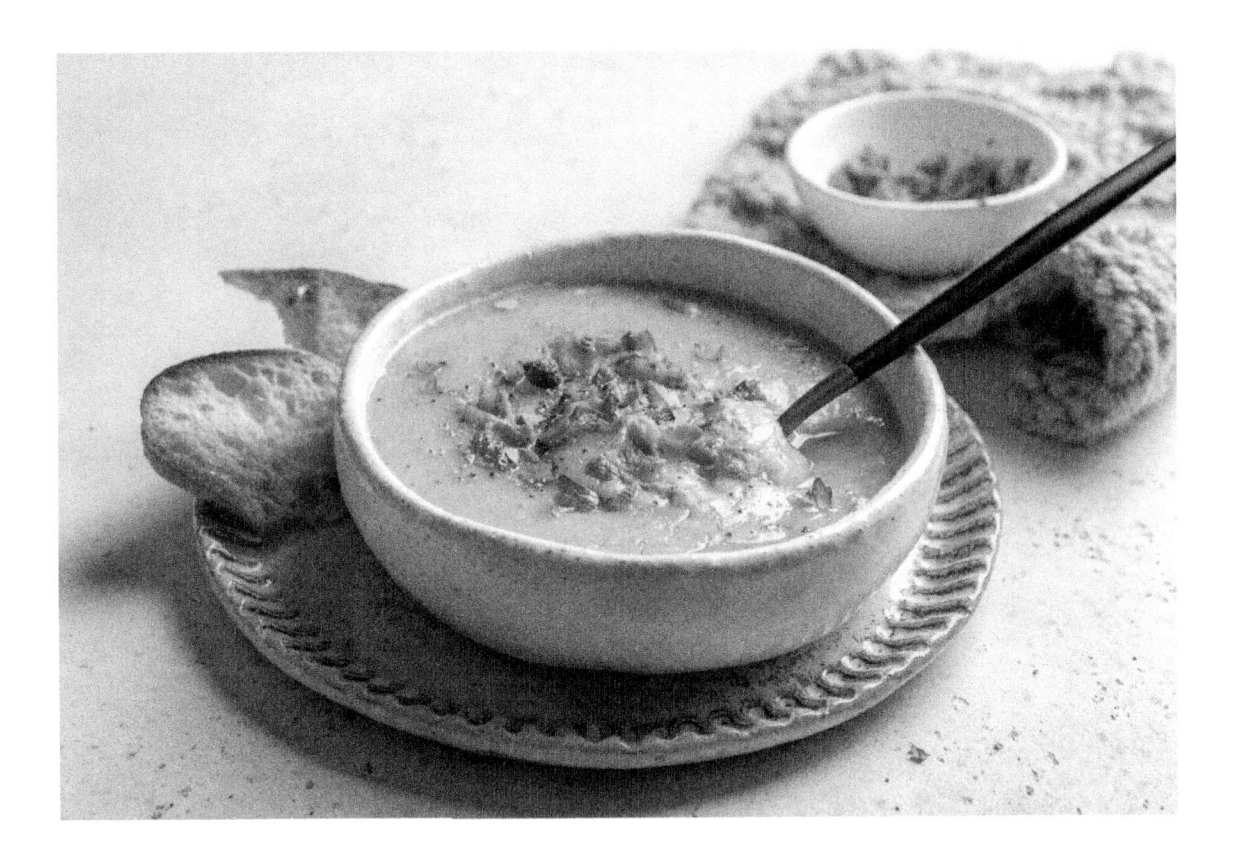

Try out on our slow cooker chorizo pea recipe with loads of nutrients to make you feel energized. The meal tastes great when raw smoky, spicy chorizo is used. However, you can substitute the chorizo with Italian sausage.

Preparation time: 4 hours **Number of servings:** 4

Ingredients

- 2 cups of low sodium chicken broth
- 1 cup of yellow split peas
- 2 cups of water
- ½ pound of diced potatoes
- 1 diced onion
- ¼ cup of sprouts for garnishing
- 2 medium-sized carrots, sliced
- ½ pound of chorizo
- Salt and ground black pepper
- 1 teaspoon of dried oregano
- ½ tablespoon of paprika
- 3 finely chopped garlic cloves

Preparation method

In a 6- quart slow cooker, add in the broth, potatoes, carrots, onions, garlic, oregano, water, ½ teaspoon of salt, peas, and paprika

Cook on low for 8hours or on high for 4 hours

Remove the chorizo and crumble them into a skillet

Cook them for 5 minutes on medium heat

Stir in the chorizo back in the soup, add ¼ teaspoon of pepper and some salt to taste

Garnish with sprouts and enjoy

30. Stuffed Sweet Potato with Hummus and Beans

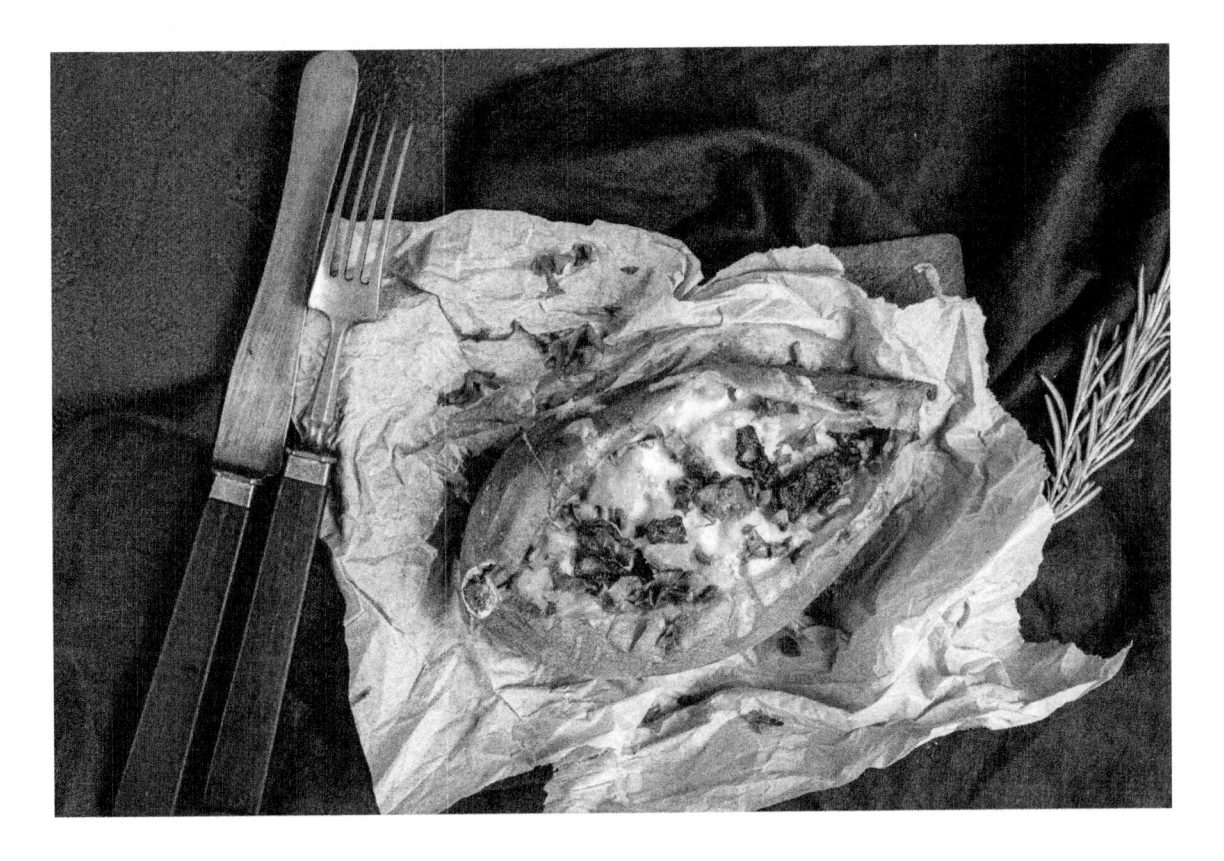

If you are looking for a simple yet hearty meal to prepare for lunch, then stuffed sweet potato with hummus and beans will be great. This protein-rich meal with hummus dressing and kales will be ready within 20 minutes.

Preparation time: 20 minutes **Number of servings:** 1

Ingredients

- ¾ cup of chopped kale
- 1 sweet potato
- ¼ cup of hummus
- 2 tablespoons of water
- 1 cup of rinsed black beans

Preparation method

Use a fork to prick the potato, microwave on high for about 10 minutes until it is cooked through

Over medium-high heat, cook the kales in a saucepan until they wilt, add in the beans, 2 tablespoons of water and cook stir for about 2 minutes

In a bowl, combine the hummus and 2 tablespoons of water or more to achieve the desired consistency

Halve the sweet potato, top with bean and kale mixture, drizzle with hummus dressing and serve

Conclusion

Eating healthy will help to lower the risk of cancer. You can achieve this by eating cruciferous vegetables, such as broccoli, kale, cauliflower, that are full of vitamin C, K, and manganese. Consumption of fish, nuts, legumes, and fruits is also beneficial to the body.

Our recipes will provide you with the nutrients that you need to help you fight cancer. Try them and enjoy.

About the Author

Molly Mills always knew she wanted to feed people delicious food for a living. Being the oldest child with three younger brothers, Molly learned to prepare meals at an early age to help out her busy parents. She just seemed to know what spice went with which meat and how to make sauces that would dress up the blandest of pastas. Her creativity in the kitchen was a blessing to a family where money was tight and making new meals every day was a challenge.

Molly was also a gifted athlete as well as chef and secured a Lacrosse scholarship to Syracuse University. This was a blessing to her family as she was the first to go to college and at little cost to her parents. She took full advantage of her college education and earned a business degree. When she graduated, she joined her culinary skills and business acumen into a successful catering business. She wrote her first e-book after a customer asked if she could pay for several of her recipes. This sparked the entrepreneurial spirit in Mills and she thought if one person wanted them, then why not share the recipes with the world!

Molly lives near her family's home with her husband and three children and still cooks for her family every chance she gets. She plays Lacrosse with a local team made up of her old teammates from college and there are always some tasty nibbles on the ready after each game.

Don't Miss Out!

Scan the QR-Code below and you can sign up to receive emails whenever Molly Mills publishes a new book. There's no charge and no obligation.

Sign Me Up

https://molly.gr8.com

Printed in Great Britain
by Amazon